IDENTIFICATION OF MICRORNA
IN *PENICILLIUM MARNEFFEI*

CHOW WANG NGAI
Ph. D. THESIS

THE UNIVERSITY OF HONG KONG
2013

Abstract of thesis entitled

"Identification of microRNA

in *Penicillium marneffei*"

Submitted by

CHOW Wang Ngai

for the degree of Doctor of Philosophy

at The University of Hong Kong

in March 2013

Penicillium marneffei is the most important thermal dimorphic fungus causing respiratory, skin and systemic mycosis in China and Southeast Asia. While miRNAs are increasingly recognized for their roles in post-transcriptional regulation of gene expression in animals and plants, the existence of miRNAs in fungi was less well studied and their potential roles in fungal dimorphism were largely unknown. Based on available genome sequence of *P. marneffei*, it is hypothesized that miRNA-like small RNAs (milRNAs) may be expressed in the dimorphic fungus and dicer- or argonuate-like proteins may be involved in dimorphism or virulence in *P. marneffei*.

I attempted to identify milRNAs in *P. marneffei* in both mycelial and yeast phase using high-throughput sequencing technology. Small RNAs were more abundantly expressed in mycelial than yeast phase. Sequence analysis revealed 24 potential milRNA candidates, including 17 (2502 reads) candidates in mycelial and seven (232 reads) in yeast phase. Two genes, *dcl-1* and *dcl-2*, encoding putative Dicer-like proteins and the gene, *qde-2*, encoding Argonaute-like protein, were identified in *P. marneffei*. Phylogenetic analysis showed that *dcl-2* and *qde-2* of *P. marneffei* were more closely related to the homologues in the thermal dimorphic pathogenic fungi, *Histoplasma capsulatum*, *Blastomyces dermatitidis*, *Paracoccidioides brasiliensis* and *Coccidioides immitis* than to *Penicillium chrysogenum* and *Aspergillus* spp., suggesting the co-evolution of *dcl-2* and *qde-2* among other thermal dimorphic fungi. Moreover, *dcl-2* and *qde-2* demonstrated higher mRNA expression levels in mycelial than yeast phase by 7 folds and 2 folds respectively ($P<0.001$). Northern blot analysis confirmed the expression of two milRNAs, *PM-milR-M1* and *PM-milR-M2*, only in mycelial phase. Using $dcl-1^{KO}$, $dcl-2^{KO}$, dcl^{DKO} and $qde-2^{KO}$ deletion mutants, it was shown that the biogenesis of both milRNAs were dependent on *dcl-2* but not *dcl-1* or *qde-2*. While deletion of *qde-2*, but not the two *dcl* genes, was found to decrease the virulence level of *P. marneffei* in mice model, the deaths of the $qde-2^{KO}$ conidia challenged mice were delayed for over 10 days. The $qde-2^{KO}$ conidia have lower recovery rate both in human THP1 and murine J774 macrophage cell lines and also reduced resistance to hydrogen peroxide than the wild type.

This study provided the first evidence for differential expression of milRNAs in different growth phases of thermal dimorphic fungi and shed light on the evolution of fungal proteins involved in milRNA biogenesis and possible role of post-transcriptional control in governing thermal dimorphism. This is also the first study to reveal the relationship between argonuate-like QDE-2 protein and virulence in *P. marneffei* in mice model. This study provides a foundation for the milRNAs study in pathogenic thermal dimorphic fungi.

-   An abstract of exactly 425 words   -

Identification of microRNA
in *Penicillium marneffei*

Thesis submitted for the degree of Doctor of Philosophy

at The University of Hong Kong

by

CHOW Wang Ngai

B.Sc. (2005), M. Phil. (2007), HKU

Department of Microbiology

The Univesity of Hong Kong

March 2013

DECLARATION

I, CHOW Wang Ngai, declare that this thesis represents my own work, except where

due acknowledgement is made, and that it has not been previously included in a thesis,

dissertation or report submitted to this University or to any other institution for a

degree, diploma or other qualifications.

_____

CHOW Wang Ngai

CONJOINT WORK

The following publication contains materials that are also included in this thesis, and I declare that I have been responsible for the contributions to the publication as listed.

_____

CHOW Wang Ngai

1. Woo, P.C., S.K. Lau, B. Liu, J.J. Cai, K.T. Cheong, H. Tse, R.Y. Kao, C.M. Chan, **W.N. Chow**, K.Y. Yuen. 2011. Draft genome sequence of _Penicillium marneffei_ strain PM1. Eukaryot Cell 10(12):1740-1

2. Lau S. K. P., **W.N. Chow** (co-first author), A.Y.P. Wong, J.M.Y. Yeung, J. Bao, N. Zhang, S. Lok, P.C.Y. Woo, K.Y. Yuen. 2013. Identification of microRNA-like RNAs in mycelial and yeast phases of the thermal dimorphic fungus _Penicillium marneffei_. 2013. PLOS Neglected Tropical Diseases (under revision)

ii

ACKNOWLEDGEMENTS

None of this would have been possible without the generous help of many people in The University of Hong Kong. I would like to express my gratitude to all of my teachers, especially my supervisors Dr. Susanna K. P. Lau and Prof. Kwok-Yung Yuen for their enlightenment, encouragement and guidance for my studies. I would also like to thank Prof. Patrick C.Y. Woo who shared his invaluable advice and knowledge with me. I am grateful to Prof. Si Lok, Jessie Bao and Na Zhang for their collaboration and expertise in performing Illuminia/Solexa Sequencing.

Many thanks to my friends and colleagues for their support and technical assistance over the past years, including Annette Wong, Juilian Yeung and Tom Ho for their valuable suggestion in bioinformatics and members in the Department of Microbiology especially Candy Lau, Chris Tsang, Cyril Yip, George Lo, H.W. Tsoi, Jade Teng, Philip Yeung, Shirly Curreem, Wendy Yang and, in particular, Apple Leung, Edward Tung and Emily Tam for their continuous support during all the time.

Last but not least, I would like to thank my father H.W. Chow, my mother Anita W.S. Cheung (1949-2012) and my sister Elaine Y.L. Chow for their love, caring and unconditional support and encouragement throughout my life. May the soul of my dearest mother rest in peace.

CONTENTS

CHAPTER 2 MATERIALS AND METHODS

CHAPTER 3 FUNCTIONAL CHARACTERIZATION OF DCL-1, DCL-2 AND QDE-2 PROTEINS

CHAPTER 4 IDENTIFICATION OF NOVEL MICRORNA-LIKE RNA IN *P. MARNEFFEI*

LIST OF FIGURES

xi

LIST OF TABLES

ABBREVIATIONS

AIDS	Acquired immunodeficiency syndrome
BHI	Brain Heart Infusion
BLAST	Basic Local Alignment Search Tool
CFU	Colony forming unit
CoA	Coenzyme A
DIG	Digoxigenin
DNA	Deoxyribonucleic Acid
DNase	Deoxyribonuclease
dNTP	Deoxynucleoside triphosphate
dsRNA	Double stranded RNA
EDTA	Ethylene diaminetetra-acetic acid
HAART	Highly active antiretroviral therapy
HBSS	Hank's buffered salt solution
HIV	Human immunodeficiency virus
IFN-γ	Interferon gamma
ITS	Internal transcribed spacer regions
MEGA	Molecular evolutionary genetics analysis
MOI	Multiplicity of infection
MUSCLE	Multiple sequence comparison by log-expectation

miRNA	Micro-RNA
mRNA	Messenger RNA
NCBI	National Center for Biotechnology Information
PBS	Phosphate buffered saline
PCR	Polymerase chain reaction
PEG	Polyethylene glycol
RPMI	Roswell Park Memorial Institute medium
PKS	Polyketide synthase
PTGS	Post transcriptional gene silencing
RISC	RNA induced silencing complex
RNA	Ribonucleic acid
RNAi	RNA interference
rRNA	Ribosomal RNA
siRNA	Small interfering RNA
SDS	Sodium dodecyl sulfate
TE buffer	Tris-EDTA buffer
Th	T helper
TNF-α	Tumor necrosis factor α
Tris	Tris(hydroxymethyl)aminomethane
YPD	Yeast Peptone Dextrose

SYMBOLS

%	Percent
°C	Degree Celsius
bp	Base pair
g	Gram
h	Hour
kb	Kilo base pair
M	Molar
min	Minute
ml	Milliliter
mM	Millimolar
no	Number
β	Beta
μg	Microgram
μl	Microliter
μM	Micromolar
μm	Micrometer

CHAPTER 1 INTRODUCTION

1.1 *P. marneffei*

1.1.1 *P. marneffei* as an emerging pathogen

Fungi are ubiquitous microorganisms in our daily living. They are widely used for antibiotic production, such as penicillin, or served as food substances. Most fungi are considered clinically unimportant and they do not pose threat to human health. However, some fungi can cause opportunistic infection to human. Fungal pathogens infect human with primary or acquired immunodeficiency as a result of radiotherapy, chemotherapy, hematological disorders or human immunodeficiency virus (HIV) infection (Guarro, GeneJ et al. 1999).

Although *Penicillium* species are usually considered as non-pathogenic, *P. marneffei* is different. *P. marneffei*, the only thermal dimorphic fungus under the genus *Pencillium*, is an opportunistic fungal pathogen. It infects immunocompromised patients particularly HIV-positive patients. *P. marneffei* was firstly isolated from the liver of *Rhizomys sinensis* (bamboo rat) in 1956. It was named after the director of the Pasteur Institute of Indochina and Paris incumbent, Dr. Hubert Marneffe during the time of discovery (Capponi, Segretain et al. 1956). The disease that is caused by *P. marneffei* is called penicilliosis. Penicilliosis was firstly reported in 1959 as a laboratory acquired infection in human (Segretain 1959). The first case of naturally occurring human penicilliosis was reported much later in a patient with Hodgkin's disease (DiSalvo, Fickling et al. 1973). Penicilliosis was once considered as a rarely occurred disease, with only 18 cases reported between 1956 and 1988. Until the late 1980s, that the spread of HIV-AIDS

1

pandemic came to Southeast Asia (Deng, Ribas et al. 1988), *P. marneffei* infections have become endemic in Vietnam (Huynh, Nguyen et al. 2003), China (Deng, Ribas et al. 1988; Luh 1998; Wong, Lee et al. 1998), India (Ranjana, Priyokumar et al. 2002), and Thailand where the majority cases of penicilliosis have been reported (Supparatpinyo, Chiewchanvit et al. 1992; Supparatpinyo, Khamwan et al. 1994). Other countries with reported penicilliosis cases include Cambodia (Sar, Boy et al. 2006), Malaysia and Myanmar (Kaldor, Sittitrai et al. 1994). Some HIV patients who had visited endemic countries were also infected by *P. marneffei* when they returned to their home countries. However, cases of penicilliosis are rare in other parts of the world.

1.1.2 Mycology

1.1.2.1 Taxonomy

Fungi were under the Plant Kingdom in past. However, scientists later on discovered distinctive difference between the fungal cells and the plant cells. Plant cells possess cellulose cell walls but fungal cells contain chitin cell walls. Moreover, in plants, zygotoes develop into diploid and evolve into multicellularities, while in fungi, zygotoes undergo meiosis and most of the vegetative phases are in haploid. In addition, plants are autotrophs that undergo photosynthesis with the present of chloroplast but fungi are heterotrophs and saprotrophs (Kendrick 2001).

In 1969, Robert Harding Whittaker proposed fungi, which were previously classified as plants, should be given their own kingdom. Thus, fungi were classified into a separate kingdom belonging to the *Eukaryota* domain (Jahn, Bovee et al. 1979). Fungi were further divided into eight phyla mainly according to their reproductive characteristics: *Ascomycota, Basidiomycota, Blastocladiomycota, Chytridiomycota, Cryptomycota, Glomeromycota, Microsporidia* and *Neocallimastigomycota*. The phyla of *Ascomycota* and *Basidiomycota* were grouped into the subkingdom of *Dikarya* (Hibbett, Binder et al. 2007) (NCBI, Taxonomy 2012/6/7)).

Penicillium is under the phyla of *Ascomycota*. Ascomycetes in teleomorph stages (sexual reproductive stages) produce ascospores (asci) inside their reproductive structures. While in anamorph stages (asexual reproductive stages), ascomycetes produce conidia. In the life cycles of ascomycetes, most of their times remain as anamorphs and most of ascomycetes do not have teleomorphs. *P.*

marneffei belongs to the subphylum *Pezizomycotina* (James, Kauff et al. 2006), the class *Eurotiomycetes*, the order *Eurotiales*, the family *Trichocomaceae* and the genus *Penicillium* (Kendrick 2000). *Penicillium* is under subgenus of *Biverticillium*. Phylogenetic analysis of *Penicillium* species, based on ribosomal RNA gene sequencing, reveals *Talaromyces* are the closest sexual species related to *Penicillium*. Therefore, *Penicillium* species are thought to be the anamorphs of *Talaromyces* species (LoBuglio and Taylor 1995). Until 2011, the review by Samson *et al.* suggested that *P. marneffei* should be classified under *Talaromyces* instead of *Penicillium*. They reviewed that *Biverticillium* is phylogenetically closer with *Talaromyces* species than to other subgenera in *Penicillium*, according to the gene sequences from RPB1 (RNA polymerase II largest subunit), small subunit (SSU) rRNA, large subunit (LSU) rRNA and internal transcribed spacer regions (ITS) (Samson, Yilmaz et al. 2011).

P. marneffei was once claimed to be the most asexual ascomycetes ever known (Fisher, Hanage et al. 2005). However, in 2006, most of the sexual cycle related meiotic and mating genes were found in the genome of *P. marneffei*. This discovery turned to a possibility that mating form of *P. marneffei* is yet to be discovered (Woo, Chong et al. 2006). Further investigation into the genome could provide further information to support the possibility of the existence of the sexual form in *P. marneffei*.

1.1.2.2 Thermal dimorphism of *P. marneffei*

According to the morphology, fungi can be classified as yeast or mould. The

4

total number of fungal species is estimated to be over 5.1 million in the world (Blackwell 2011). Despite the huge numbers of fungal species, only six of the species are found to be thermal dimorphic. They are *Blastomyces dermatitidis*, *Coccidiodes immitis*, *Histoplasma capsulatum*, *Paracoccidioides brasiliensis*, *P. marneffei* and *Sporothrix schenckii*. Thermal dimorphic fungi exist in saprophytic mould phase at 25°C and in pathogenic yeast phase during 37°C (body temperature of most mammals). The mechanism of reversible phase transition in fungi is commonly believed to be regulated by unknown signal transduction pathways (Sanchez-Martinez and Perez-Martin 2001). Recent years, a histidine kinase, DRK1, was reported to be the global switches controlling dimorphic in *B. dermatitidis* and *H. capsulatum* (Nemecek, Wuthrich et al. 2006). However, in *P. marneffei*, some genes have been studied regarding the morphogenetic circuitry, but no real dimorphic switch is discovered yet. Under the *Eurotiales* order and the *Penicillium* genus, *P. marneffei* is the only thermal dimorphic fungus. There are three homothallic forms in the life cycle of *P. marneffei*: during 25°C, it exists as (I) filamentous vegetative form, (II) asexual conidial form and at 37°C, it appears as (III) arthroconidial yeast like form (Figure 1).

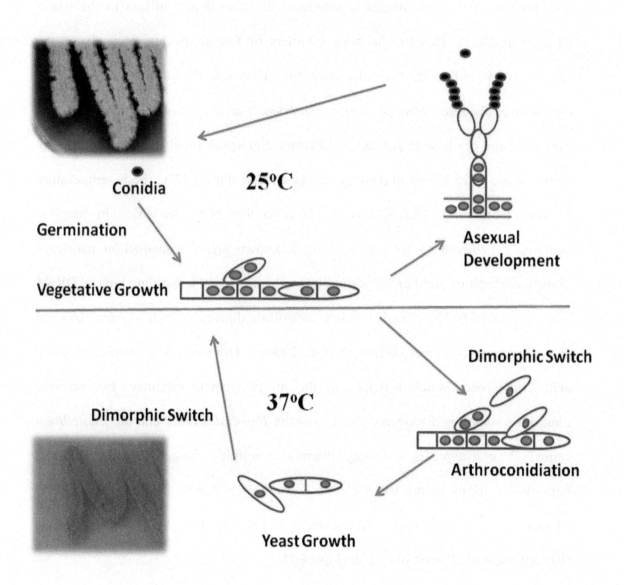

Figure 1. Dimorphism of *P. marneffei*. *P. marneffei* grown in mold and yeast phases on Sabouraud dextrose agar.

1.1.2.3 Mould phase of *P. marneffei*

P. marneffei exists as mould at 25°C, with the production of uninucleate conidia. A conidium germinates under suitable conditions. It expands isotopically to produce germ tube. Hypha is produced by the polarized elongation growth of the germ tube. Septa is then formed to separate the cellular compartments behind the apical tip. There are multiple nuclei inside the growing cellular compartments. The older subapical cells are usually uninucleate. Repolarizing of subapical cells is carried out to produce elongating branched cells (Kavanagh 2007).

In the asexual reproduction of *P. marneffei*, the conidiophore undergoes conidiogenesis to produce conidia (2-3μm diameter) (Andrianopoulos 2002; Kavanagh 2007). In the presence of nutrient and air interface, conidiogenesis starts after hyphae formation at 25°C. Laboratory culture of *P. marneffei* on solid growth medium with an air interface leads to conidiogenesis, while conidiation occurs rarely in shaking liquid culture broth (Andrianopoulos 2002; Cooper and Vanittanakom 2008).

P. marneffei secretes water soluble brick red pigment (in solid and liquid media) and produces yellow conidia in mould phase (in solid medium). Under the genus *Penicillium*, *P. citrinum*, *P. janthinellum* and *P. rubrum* also produce diffusible red pigment. However, these three species are not pathogenic fungi. Therefore, the red pigment of *P. marneffei* is the key identity for clinical diagnosis (Bhardwaj, Shukla et al. 2007).

1.1.2.4 Yeast phase of *P. marneffei*

P. marneffei exists as yeast form (reproduced by fission) at 37°C. The conidia germinate to produce highly branched uninucleate hyphae like cells called pre-arthroconidial cells with about 20 μm in length, which is about half the length of the vegetative hyphal cells (~40 μm) in the mould phase. Double septa separate the cellular compartments of the multicellular pre-arthroconidia. Then uninucleate arthroconidia are formed by the degradation of double septa. Yeast cells (3-8 μm) are produced by arthroconidia by fission (Andrianopoulos 2002; Kavanagh 2007).

No red pigment is produced in the yeast phase of *P. marneffei*. The yeast colony appeared in white to grey color, with minor secretions of brown or tan pigment. The phenotypic difference between the two phases in *P. marneffei* is a unique and important feature that is used in clinical identification of the fungus.

1.1.2.5 Molecular genetics in *P. marneffei* morphogenesis

The morphogenetic control of conidial germination, hyphal growth, asexual development and yeast morphogenesis are governed by many genes in *P. marneffei*. Conidial germination was found to be regulated by GasC, RasA, CflA and PakA proteins. GasC, a subunit of heterotrimetric G proteins, is required for conidial germination at both 25 and 37°C to interact with receptors to transmit environmental signals. Deletion of *gasC* showed a reduction in germination in both phases than that of the wild type (Zuber, Hynes et al. 2003). RasA and CflA are Ras and Rho GTPase family proteins, which act downstream and upstream of GasC respectively. Dominant negative *rasA*^{D125A} mutant delayed the germination at 25°C (Boyce, Hynes et al. 2005) and *cflA*^{D120A} dominant negative mutant decreased germination rates in both phases (Boyce, Hynes et al. 2001). Deletion of *pakA*, gene which encodes the downstream p21-activated kinase (PAK), resulted in certain extent in reduction of germination at mycelial phase but almost completely termination in germination at yeast phase (Boyce and Andrianopoulos 2007). Morphogenetic control of hyphal growth and polarity in *P. marneffei* required Rho GTPase, CflA and CflB, and PakA and PakB. Rho has a conserved role in the regulation of actin-mediated polarization growth in fungi. While both CflA and CflB are needed for the polarized hyphal growth, but only CflB is required for polarized conidiophores growth. Mutation of both *cflA* and *cflB* showed actin could not be concentrated at the hyphal apex. *cflB* single deletion mutant resulted in malformed, hyperbranched hyphal cells (Boyce, Hynes et al. 2001; Boyce, Hynes et al. 2003). Rho GTPase regulates polarized growth not solely by actin recruitment but also by activating downstream PAKs to regulate cellular division and polarized growth. The downstreams of Rho GTPase include PakA and PakB. PakA involved in conidial germination, whereas pakB is regarded as the growth signal in the hypha at 25°C (Boyce and Andrianopoulos 2007; Boyce, Schreider et al. 2009). Conidiogenesis of *P. marneffei* occurs at 25°C to produce asexual spores (conidia). The heterotrimetric G_a subunits of GasA and GasC, and together with the downstream RasA, were found to regulate asexual development (Zuber, Hynes et al. 2002; Zuber, Hynes et al. 2003; Boyce, Hynes et al. 2005). Either *gasA*^{G203R} dominant negative or *gasC* deletion mutant increased conidiation, while overexpression of either one decreased conidiation in *P. marneffei* (Zuber, Hynes et al. 2002; Zuber, Hynes et al. 2003). Dominant negative mutant of *rasA*^{D125A} showed early initiation of conidiation (Boyce, Hynes et al. 2005).

P. marneffei undergos arthroconidiation to become uninucleate fission yeast cells when switched to 37°C. However, during infection, this process of arthroconidiation is bypassed. The pulmonary alveolar macrophages in the host phagocytosed the conidia. The conidia germinate into yeast cells intracellularly in macrophages (Vanittanakom, Cooper et al. 2006; Boyce, Schreider et al. 2011). Genes, *pakA*, *pakB*, *drkA* and *slnA* are involved in yeast morphogenesis of *P. marneffei*. Deletion of *pakA* resulted in reduction of conidial germination during macrophage infection and *in vitro*. On the other hand, those macrophages that phagocytosed the conidia of *pakB* deletion mutant showed no yeast cells exist but highly branched hyphals cells. This study suggested that PakB is needed for yeast cell division during infection (Boyce, Schreider et al. 2009). It was found that the temperature sensor hybrid histidine kinases, DrkA and SlnA, are needed for yeast growth at 37°C (Boyce, Schreider et al. 2011). Delayed conidial germination at 37°C was observed in *slnA* deletion mutant. Both *slnA* and *drkA* deletion mutants produce swollened arthroconidiating hyphal cells and fewer septa (Boyce, Schreider et al. 2011). In macrophages, deletion mutants of *slnA* or *drkA* were unable to produce yeast cells, but remained as ungerminated-conidia and mostly converted to germlings in *slnA* and *drkA* deletion mutants, respectively (Boyce, Schreider et al. 2011). Indeed, *drkA* in *P. marneffei*, which yeast is divided by fission, is conserved in both *B. dermatitidis* and *H. capsulatum*, which yeasts are divided by budding, as *drk1*. However, *drk1* is the master regulator of the dimorphic switch in *B. dermatitidis* and *H. capsulatum*, but *drkA* only regulates the dimorphism of *P. marneffei* in macrophages (Nemecek, Wuthrich et al. 2006). Although DrkA and SlnA are involved in the 37°C sensing to a downstream pathway in yeast transition of *P. marneffei*, it is still unclear which genes regulate the actual dimorphic switch in all aspects.

1.1.3   Ecology and Epidemiology of *P. marneffei*

1.1.3.1   Reservoirs and route of transmission

P. marneffei was first isolated from the liver of a bamboo rat, *R. sinensis*, in South Vietnam in 1956 (Capponi, Segretain et al. 1956). Three decades later, in 1986, another bamboo rat, *R. pruinosus,* was found to be the carrier of *P. marneffei* in Guangxi region of China (Deng, Yun et al. 1986). Later, in 1996, two more species of bamboo rats, *R. sumatrensis and Cannomys badius*, were also found to be infected with *P. marneffei* in Thailand (Chariyalertsak, Vanittanakom et al. 1996). Besides Thailand and China, *P. marneffei* were also isolated from 10% of the captured *C. babdius* in India.

Genotyping of *P. marneffei* strains that were isolated from infected patients showed that the sequences were perfectly identical to a *P. marneffei* stain isolated from wild bamboo rat. This finding raised a hypothesis for the existence of transmission between bamboo rats and humans or illustrated bamboo rats and humans were coninfected with a common source (Gugnani, Fisher et al. 2004). However, except bamboo rats, no other rodents were found to be the carriers of *P. marneffei*, even they were living in close habitats with bamboo rats. It suggested the possibility of the existence of host-specific factors for *P. marneffei* (Gugnani, Fisher et al. 2004). Nevertheless, the reasons behind remain unclear.

Several studies tried to isolate *P. marneffei* from various sources such as bamboos,

11

soil burrows of bamboo rats and soil samples from the residential areas of penicilliosis patients. However, only three soil burrow samples showed positive results and the rests were all negatives (Deng, Ribas et al. 1988; Chariyalertsak, Vanittanakom et al. 1996). In another study, which was carried out by Vanittanakom, Mekaprateep et al., demonstrated *P. marneffei* could not be recovered from environmental and sterile soil samples, suggesting the survival of *P. marneffei* was very likely to be limited by other fungal competitors. Apparently, *P. marneffei* was not originated from soil (Vanittanakom, Mekaprateep et al. 1995).

P. marneffei is believed to be transmitted through inhalation of conidia and dissemination to lung, same as the transmission route of other thermal dimorphic fungi. The acquisition of coccidiomycosis by *C. immitisis* is proven to be via breathing of the dust-borne arthroconidia when mammals are exposed to the contaminated soil (Laniado-Laborin 2007). The acquisition of acute histoplasmosis by *H. capsulatum* is caused by wind-borne spores from soil that was contaminated with bird or bat droppings containing *H. capsulatum* spores (Laniado-Laborin 2007). From the route of transmission of these endemic thermal dimorphic fungi, it is postulated that penicilliosis by *P. marneffei* is caused by the inhalation of conidia from contaminated sources such as the droppings from bamboo rats and then disseminated in the lungs of the infected immunocompromised patients. Although the suggested transmission route of *P. marneffei* is by inhalation, it is still unknown whether the transmission occurs through zoonotic (animal) or sapronotic (environmental) source or even through multiple sources. The sources of transmission of pathogens (including *P. marneffei*) are always an ongoing research topic in microbiology.

1.1.3.2 Seasonal variation of *P. marneffei* infections

Seasonal variation of penicilliosis occurs in northern Thailand (Chariyalertsak, Sirisanthana et al. 1996). A four-year study was carried out to investigate the number of *P. marneffei* infected cases and *C. neoformans* infected cases among different seasons. This study showed *P. marneffei* infections were likely to occur more frequently in the rainy season (between May and October) while there was no seasonal fluctuation can be documented in *C. neoformans* infections. Indeed, the number of immunocompromised patients was unlikely to be varied among different seasons. The seasonal variation of *P. marneffei* infection was probably related to the changes in animal reservoirs (behavior or growth conditions). It was possible that hot and wet climate promoted the growth of the bamboo rats or the growth of *P. marneffei*. As a result, more conidia were released to the environment. A larger proportion of immunocompromised patients inhaled the conidia and got infections.

1.1.3.3 Geographical variation of *P. marneffei*

Like other opportunistic pathogenic fungi, a higher incidence rate of *P. marneffei* infection in AIDS endemic areas such as Sub-Saharan Africa is expected. Surprisingly, Africa, the top most HIV-AIDS cases are documented in the world, is not an endemic area of *P. marneffei* infection, suggesting the incidence of penicilliosis does not follow the distribution of HIV-AIDS. Instead, Southeast Asia, the second most incidences in HIV, is the only endemic area of *P. marneffei* infections (UNAIDS 2007). It remains a question for the scientists to investigate and explain.

Although *P. marneffei* was discovered in Southern Vietnam, only a minor number of penicilliosis cases were reported in there (Capponi, Segretain et al. 1956). Thailand is the region where most penicilliosis were diagnosed (1,173 cases were reported at Chiang Mai University Hospital between 1991 and 1997) (Sirisanthana and Supparatpinyo 1998). In Northeastern India, one-fourth HIV-positive patients were diagnosed to have *P. marneffei* infections (Sirisanthana and Supparatpinyo 1998; Ranjana, Priyokumar et al. 2002). Penicilliosis was also documented from other Asian countries including Cambodia (Sar, Boy et al. 2006), China (Deng, Ribas et al. 1988; Luh 1998; Wong and Lee 1998), Malaysia and Myanmar (Kaldor, Sittitrai et al. 1994). Non-endemic countries including Australia (Jones and See 1992), France (Hilmarsdottir, Meynard et al. 1993), Germany (Sobottka, Albrecht et al. 1996), Italy (Viviani, Tortorano et al. 1993), the Netherlands (Hulshof, van Zanten et al. 1990), Sweden (Julander and Petrini 1997), Switzerland (Kronauer, Schar et al. 1993), the United States (Piehl, Kaplan et al. 1988) and the United Kingdom (Peto, Bull et al. 1988) were also reported to have penicilliosis cases. All the patients that were diagnosed from non-endemic countries had a travelling history to the endemic regions before, with only one exceptional case (Lo, Tintelnot et al. 2000).

In Hong Kong, the first AIDS case was reported in 1985. Five years later, the first penicilliosis case was confirmed (Low 2002). According to a surveillance study of penicilliosis in AIDS patients conducted from 1990 to 2001, around one to seven new penicilliosis cases were reported in each year. About 8% of all AIDS patients get penicillosis as an AIDS-related illness (Low 2002). In 1995, the Hong Kong Scientific Committee of the Advisory Council on AIDS included penicilliosis as one of the AIDS-indicator diseases in the HIV infection classification system (HIV/AIDS

Surveillance Office 1995). Besides HIV patients, other immunocompromised patients are also the risk group of penicilliosis.

1.1.3.4   Risk factors

According to a 10-year surveillance study on penicilliosis in Hong Kong (1994 to 2004), over 90% of *P. marneffei* infected patients were HIV-positive (Wu, Chan et al. 2008). The data were comparable with other endemic countries. Besides the penicilliosis cases were diagnosed in HIV patients, HIV-negative patients who are under immunosuppressant treatment can also be infected with penicilliosis (Cao, Chen et al. 1998; Hsueh, Teng et al. 2000). Penicilliosis cases were also reported in HIV-negative patients with Hodgkin's disease, tuberculosis, systemic lupus erythematosus, reactive hemophagocytic syndrome, haematological malignancies, transplantation, diabetes mellitus and autoimmune disease (Chim, Fong et al. 1998; Wong, Woo et al. 2001; Lupi, Tyring et al. 2005; Wu, Chan et al. 2008).

Although bamboo rat was thought to be the reservoir of *P. marneffei*, bamboo rat had little or no contact with the penicilliosis individuals. It is speculated that bamboo rat was the host rather than the reservoir (Sirisanthana and Supparatpinyo 1998). The true environmental reservoir of *P. marneffei* is yet to be revealed.

1.1.4 Pathology, pathogenesis and Immunology

1.1.4.1 Pathogenesis and pathology

P. marneffei is a primary pulmonary pathogen. *P. marneffei* infection is acquired when the patient inhales the conidia into the respiratory tract. Conidia are then attached to the surface of bronchoalveolar epithelium. Studies suggested that the processes of adhesion is facilitated by interaction with fibronectin and laminin via a sialic acid-specific lectin (Hamilton, Jeavons et al. 1998; Hamilton, Jeavons et al. 1999), or/and glycosaminoglycans (GAGs) chondroitin sulfate B, heparin, and sulfated chitosan (CP-3) (Srinoulprasert, Kongtawelert et al. 2006) on the cell membrane of epithelial cells.

The dimorphic switching of *P. marneffei* begins at 37°C after entering to the host. Conidia germinate and grow as yeast, the virulent form which targets the mononuclear phagocytic system. The yeast cells were phagocytosed or stayed in the membrane-bound vacuoles. The yeast cells can even infiltrate macrophages or stay within the cytoplasm of the pulmonary histiocytes (Deng and Connor 1985; Chan and Chow 1990; Cui, Tanaka et al. 1997; Vanittanakom, Cooper et al. 2006).

P. marneffei can replicate in mononuclear macrophages. However, macrophages also have antifungal activities which may involve to the production of reactive nitrogen/oxygen intermediates (Kudeken, Kawakami et al. 2000). Besides, neutrophils, which are abundant in circulation, were also activated to exhibit antifungal activities in the presence of proinflammatory cytokines (GM-CSF, G-CSF and IFN-γ). TNF-α and IL-8 also aid the neutrophils to inhibit the germination of the invaded conidia.

The proliferation of *P. marneffei* in histiocytes triggers cell-mediated response in the host to form histiocytic granuloma. The granuloma expands upon the deposition of cellular debris and recruitment of immune cells (neutrophils, multinucleated giant cells and lymphocytes) continue. Central necrosis occurs within the lesion when the granuloma expands to a certain size, leading to the release of *P. marneffei* into the circulation, which may invade and disseminate other organs in the host (Vanittanakom, Cooper et al. 2006).

The immunological status of the host determines the severity of penicilliosis. Immunocompetent individuals have seldom chance to develop into a disseminated infection while immunocompromised patients such as HIV-positive individuals have greater chance of progressing into a lethal disseminated infection (Deng, Ribas et al. 1988; Tsui, Ma et al. 1992; Drouhet and Ravisse 1993). *Penicilliosis marneffei* is always a fatal infection because it is often misdiagnosed as histoplasmosis or crytococcosis as they have similar clinical presentation (Pautler, Padhye et al. 1984; Deng, Ribas et al. 1988; Hilmarsdottir, Meynard et al. 1993; Viviani, Tortorano et al. 1993; Borradori, Schmit et al. 1994; Heath, Patel et al. 1995). However, cases of prolonged asymptomatic infections have also been reported (Peto, Bull et al. 1988; Jones and See 1992). Once the hosts become immunocompromised due to aging or diseases, *P. marneffei* is likely to evade the immune system, emerge and develop into disseminate penicilloisis. The immunological status of the disseminated penicilliosis patients also determines the histopathological response. Immunocompetent patients normally have a suppurative-type or granulomatous response, while immunocompromised patients usually have anergic and necrotizing response.

A suppurative-type reaction involves a cell-mediated inflammatory response (involve neutrophils and fibrin deposition), forming multiple abscesses in various organs (especially in the lungs, skins, livers and subcutaneous tissues) (Deng, Ribas et al. 1988; Duong 1996). In the granulomatous response, formation of granulomas (usually consists of epithelioid cells, giant cells, histiocytes, lymphocytes and plasma cells) are mainly limited to organs of the mononuclear phagocytic system (primary and secondary lymphoid organs: bone marrow and thymus; lymph nodes, tonsils, spleen, respectively). On the other hand, immunocompromised patients often acquire the anergic and necrotizing response, which is characterized by a diffuse infiltration of histiocytes saturated with proliferating yeast cells, in lungs, liver and skin (Deng, Ribas et al. 1988; Supparatpinyo, Chiewchanvit et al. 1992; Tsui, Ma et al. 1992). It is believed that *P. marneffei* is released to extracellular cavity upon necrosis, leading to progression and dissemination of penicilliosis.

1.1.4.2 Immunology

1.1.4.2.1 Innate immunity against *P. marneffei*

Phagocytes are the first line of immune defense against *P. marneffei* infections; they include monocytes, macrophages, neutrophils, mast cells and dendritic cells. Human and murine macrophage cell lines were demonsrated to have phagocytic and anti-fungal activities against *P. marneffei* (Cogliati, Roverselli et al. 1997; Kudeken, Kawakami et al. 1999; Taramelli, Brambilla et al. 2000). In murine model, Toll-like receptor 2 and dectin-1 are receptors that are responsible for detecting *P. marneffei* and subsequently

18

activate dendritic cells (Nakamura, Miyazato et al. 2008). Also, nitric oxide synthase in immune cells produce an important antifungal agent - nitric oxide, when the cells are stimulated by cytokines such as interferon gamma (IFN-γ) (Cogliati, et al., 1997). Furthermore, the lysosomal activity of IFN-γ in macrophage are stimulated and then numerous pro-inflammatory cytokines are recruited to act against fungal infection (Schroder, Hertzog et al. 2004). Besides, peripheral blood mononuclear cells produce more tumor necrosis factor α (TNF-α) upon *P. marneffei* infection (Rongrungruang and Levitz 1999). Moreover, granulocyte cytokines have the abilities to inhibit conidia germination and dimorphic switching of *P. marneffei* in primary human granulocytes (Kudeken, Kawakami et al. 1999). Macrophage colony-stimulating factor (M-CSF) promotes phagocytosis and respiratory burst in monocyte-derived macrophages (Rongrungruang and Levitz, 1999). T helper (Th) response is also involved in the defense against *P. marneffei* infection: macrophages and neutrophils activations require Th-1 cells whereas Th-2 cells work antagonistically to hinder Th-1 maturation and to deactivate phagocytes.

1.1.4.2.2 Adaptive immunity against *P. marneffei*

T cells, especially CD4+, are responsible for *P. marneffei* clearance in murine models (Kudeken, Kawakami et al. 1996; Kudeken, Kawakami et al. 1997). Leukocytes, such as T-cells, are observed in the lungs of infected mice during *P. marneffei* infection (Kudeken, Kawakami et al. 1997). *P. marneffei* infection predominantly occurs in AIDS patients, because T-cell depletion is a common phenomenon among HIV patients.

19

1.1.4.3 Toxins, virulence factor and immunogenic proteins

P. marneffei is released from histocytes after necrosis, then disseminates and invades the host organs and tissues. Toxins or enzymes are produced by the fungal pathogen to cause cytotoxic effect or facilitate the growth and spread of the pathogen. It is unknown that whether *P. marneffei* secret toxins or not. However, there are five potential virulence factors and one potential immunogenic protein related to the pathogenesis in *P. marneffei*.

Histidine kinase is related to sporulation, growth and cell wall integrity of *P. marneffei* (Wang, Tao et al. 2009). Catalase-peroxidase (cepA) is an antioxidant in *A. fumigatus* and acts as virulence factor (Shibuya, Paris et al. 2006). The cepA is highly expressed in the yeast form of *P. marneffei*; thus it may aid the survival of *P. marneffei* inside host cells. Superoxide dismutase (SOD) is a virulence factor in *P. brasiliensis* (Tavares, Silva et al. 2005) and *C. neoformans* (Cox, Harrison et al. 2003), protecting the fungi against extracellular superoxide and helping the fungi to survive inside macrophages. In the yeast form of *P. marneffei* as well as during macrophage infection, sodA gene, that encodes the copper zinc superoxide dismutase, is highly expressed, suggesting its potential role in virulence (Pongpom, Cooper et al. 2005; Thirach, Cooper et al. 2007). Glyceraldehyde-3-phosphate dehydrogenase (GAPDH) and isocitrate lyase, the key enzymes involved in glycolysis and glyoxylate cycle respectively, were suggested to be potential virulence factors in *P. marneffei*. Isocitrate lyase was upregulated after internalization of macrophage, while the GAPDH expression was downregulated in yeast phase and after macrophage infection. It was suggested that GAPDH and isocitrate lyase

20

cooperate for the survival of *P. marneffei* in the glucose-deficient intracellular environment (Canovas and Andrianopoulos 2006; Thirach, Cooper et al. 2008). Although these potential virulence factors are involved in the survival of the fungus inside the host, none of them has solid proof to be virulence factors under Koch's postulate.

Mp1p, an immunogenic protein of *P. marneffei*, is a cell wall mannoprotein. The gene *mp1* which encodes Mp1p was first cloned and characterized in 1998 (Cao, Chan et al. 1998). Mp1p is abundant in *P. marneffei* and it is a potential biomarker for diagnosis of *P. marneffei* infections (Cao, Chen et al. 1998). Two Mp1p antigen capture ELISAs derived from the yeast *Pichia pastoris* expression system (Mab-Mab pair and Pabs-Mabs pair) were developed and could be used in routine diagnosis of penicilliosis with high detection sensitivity approaching 100% (Wang, Cai et al. 2011). `

1.1.5   Treatment and Prevention of penicilliosis

P. marneffei infection is an undeniably fatal disease if untreated. *P. marneffei* was demonstrated to be sensitive to itraconazole, voriconazole, ketoconazole, amphotericin B and flucytosine (Sar, Boy et al. 2006; Supparatpinyo and Schlamm 2007). The conventional approach for the treatment of penicilliosis is intravenous amphotericin B for two weeks and followed by oral itraconazole for 10 weeks (Sirisanthana, Supparatpinyo et al. 1998). Almost all HIV patients respond to this treatment with no serious adverse effect and the survival rate is over 80%. However, it is common that the infection relapses in 57% patients after completion of the conventional treatment (Supparatpinyo, Nelson et al. 1993). It is suggested that oral itraconazole is effective in secondary prophylaxis to avoid the relapses of penicilliosis as none of the patients relapses (Supparatpinyo, Chiewchanvit et al. 1992; Sirisanthana and Supparatpinyo 1998; Sirisanthana, Supparatpinyo et al. 1998). The recent standard treatment of penicilliosis is 14 days of intravenous amphotericin B followed by 400 mg/day oral itraconazole for 10 weeks, then oral itraconazole as secondary prophylaxis (Ustianowski, Sieu et al. 2008). Secondary prophylaxis is suggested to be discontinued if the patient is undergoing highly active antiretroviral therapy (HAART) and has a CD4+ T-cell count of 100 cells/mm^3 or above for 6 months (Chaiwarith, Charoenyos et al. 2007). The alternative treatment against penicilliosis is intravenous injection or oral intake of voriconazole for a maximum period of 12 weeks, with a respond rate of 88.9% (Supparatpinyo and Schlamm 2007).

Prophylaxis is a better approach than treatments after relapses in immunocompromised patients (especially HIV-positive). Chemoprophylaxis on penicillosis is being developed and the research of vaccine protection is in progress. Chemoprophylaxis has been suggested in prevention of various fungal infections in HIV patients. Itraconazole has been suggested to reduce the incidence of cryptococcosis and penicilliosis in HIV-positive patients (Chariyalertsak, Supparatpinyo et al. 2002). However, prophylaxis is not associated with a better survival rate of HIV patients, but a better life quality may be archived. Thus, chemoprophylaxis is suggested to HIV-positive patients who are going to travel to the endemic region (Perlman and Carey 2006).

The immunogenic protein, Mp1p, of *P. marneffei* is found to be a potential vaccine target against penicilliosis. It has been demonstrated (Wong, Woo et al. 2002) MP1 DNA vaccine was fully protective (100%) in a mouse model against intravenous challenge with *P. marneffei* yeast. While only 40% survival was observed in mice that received MP1 recombinant protein vaccine. The effectiveness of MP1 DNA vaccine requires further evaluation in different animal models before real-life application.

1.1.6 Genome of *P. marneffei*

The availability of genome data of different pathogens enables scientists to investigate their pathogenicity via bioinformatic approach. Virulence factors and genes of important pathways could be revealed through the genome studies. Currently, there are two draft genomes of *P. marneffei* strains available in Genbank: *P. marneffei ATCC 18224* and *P. marnefffei PM1*.

The Institute for Genomic Research - TIGR (Now J. Craig Venter Institute) published a draft genome of *P. marneffei ATCC 18224* strain (isolated from a Chinese bamboo rat in Vietnam) in 2007, with 8.6×coverage, 28,643,865 consensus bases, 589 contigs [Genbank: ABAR00000000.1].

In 2002, our research group collaborated with the Beijing Genome Institute on the *P. marneffei* Genome Project using strain PM1, isolated from a patient in Hong Kong, with 6×coverage of the draft genome, which has enabled the study of its mitochondrial genome sequence and revealed genomic evidence for a potential sexual cycle of *P. marneffei* (Woo, Zhen et al. 2003; Woo, Chong et al. 2006). The draft genome of PM1 consists of 2,780 sequence contigs with a total length of 28,887,485 bp and a G+C content of 47% (Woo, Lau et al. 2011) [Genbank:AGCC00000000.1].

However, as the traditional Sanger sequencing technique for fungal genome sequencing is very expensive and time consuming, no complete *P. marneffei* genome sequence (estimated genome size ~28Mb) is currently available, which has drastically hindered studies of its biology and pathogenesis by functional genomics and proteomics. It is hoped that the next generation deep sequencing systems could speed up and reduce the cost of pathogenic fungal genome sequencing to benefit pathogenicity research.

1.2   MicroRNAs

1.2.1   MicroRNAs

MicroRNAs are a class of regulatory small non-coding RNAs, with about 22 nucleotides in length (Lee and Ambros 2001). The position 2-7 or 2-8 nucleotides sequences from the 5' terminal are the seed region that is important for target recognition in animals (Kiriakidou, Nelson et al. 2004; Brennecke, Stark et al. 2005; Aleman, Doench et al. 2007). MicroRNAs regulate target gene expression by inducing mRNA cleavage or translational repression in a posttranscriptional manner (Lee, Feinbaum et al. 2004).

MicroRNAs have been identified in most eukaryotes such as plants (Reinhart, Weinstein et al. 2002), animals (Lau, Lim et al. 2001; Lagos-Quintana, Rauhut et al. 2002; Lim, Glasner et al. 2003), algae (Molnar, Schwach et al. 2007; Odling-Smee 2007), social amoeba (Hinas, Reimegard et al. 2007) and fungi (Lee, Li et al. 2010), regulating genes that involve in development, proliferation, differentiation, cell fate determination, apoptosis, signal transduction, organ development, host-viral interactions and diseases (Guarnieri and DiLeone 2008; Bartel 2009).

1.2.1.1 Discovery of miRNAs

MicroRNA (miRNA) was named in 2001 (Lau, Lim et al. 2001; Lee and Ambros 2001) and discovered by Victor Ambros, Rosalind Lee and Rhonda Feinbaum during the study of lin-4 gene of *C. elegans* in 1993. They found that lin-4 gene was vital for the developmental events in *C. elegans*. However, its open reading frame did not encode any protein. The gene was transcribed into two short transcripts (22nt and 61nt) that were antisense to the 3' UTR regions of lin-14 mRNA (Lee, Feinbaum et al. 1993). It was believed that this tiny RNA regulatory event was only an idiosyncrasy of nematode. After seven years, the second tiny regulatory RNA was identified from the let-7 gene in *C. elegans*. Surprisingly, the let-7 gene expression level greatly influenced the developmental stages (both larval and adult) in *C. elegans*. The short RNA transcript of let-7 gene targeted multiple genes (lin-14, lin-28, lin-41, lin-42 and daf-12) rather than single gene (Reinhart, Slack et al. 2000). Small RNA from let-7 was found to be conserved among varies animal species (vertebrate, ascidians, hemichordate, mollusk, annelid and arthropod), indicating a common conserved event across species (Pasquinelli, Reinhart et al. 2000), After all, research field and nomenclature on microRNA have been started (Lagos-Quintana, Rauhut et al. 2001; Lau, Lim et al. 2001; Lee and Ambros 2001).

1.2.1.1.1 MicroRNA and siRNA

The two famous classes of regulatory RNA interference (RNAi) small RNAs are microRNA and siRNA (small interference RNAs); they are similar in several aspects: (I) average size is about 21-22nt in length; (II) function as Post-Transcriptional Gene Silencing (PTGS); (III) generated by same mechanisms, processed by Dicers including the characteristic 5' phosphate groups and 2 nt overhangs on their 3'ends (Nykanen, Haley et al. 2001; Martinez, Patkaniowska et al. 2002).

siRNA can be exogenous or endogenous depending on its origin. Exogenous siRNA could be: A) A synthetic molecule that is transfected into cells in order to reduce the expression of target genes or B) Exogenous viral dsRNA, which is originated from virus replication intermediates. It is an antiviral mechanism in plants, *Drosophila* (Lagos-Quintana, Rauhut et al. 2001; Katiyar-Agarwal, Morgan et al. 2006) and mammalian cells (Ruby, Jan et al. 2006). Endogenous siRNAs (endo-siRNAs) have been discovered in plants and animals (Ambrose, Onders et al. 2001; Pallini, Pierconti et al. 2001). They are originated from long dsRNA (from antisence transcripts, pseudogenes, repetitive elements and inverted repeats) to mediate gene silencing events (Figure 2).

In fungi, siRNA transcripts usually come from repetitive sequences in transposable elements to defend against viral particles (in the chestnut blight fungus *Cryphonectria parasitica*) (Ambrose, Onders et al. 2001) and transposon invasion. Moreover, siRNA in *Neurospora crassa* maintains the genome integrity by suppressing chromosomal rearrangements events during mitosis (quelling) or silencing unpaired DNA/chromosome during the sexual cycle (meiotic silencing of unpaired DNA, MSUD) (Sun, Choi et al. 2009; Dang, Yang et al. 2011).

The major difference between miRNA and siRNA is the structure of their precursors. The precursor of miRNA is a single-stranded hairpin shaped RNA whereas siRNA is generated by a long double-stranded RNA. Moreover, mature siRNA is usually perfectly complementary to the particular target mRNA, destabilizing the target mRNA. Nonetheless, miRNA could be imperfectly (in animals) or almost perfectly complementary (in plants) to the target mRNA, resulting in translational repression or target degradation (Katiyar-Agarwal, Morgan et al. 2006; Ruby, Jan et al. 2006).

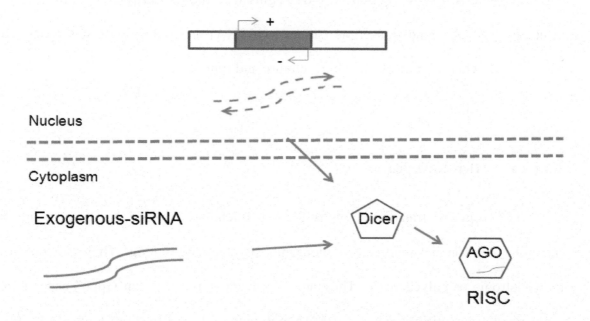

Figure 2. Exogenous and endogenous siRNA biogenesis pathway. Exogenous or endogenous dsRNAs are processed by Dicer protein and binded to AGO protein, forming the RISC for post-transcriptional gene regulation.

1.2.1.2 Biogenesis of miRNA

Biogenesis of tiny 21-24nt miRNA begins with the transcription of miRNA genes in eukaryotes. The long transcripts (primary-miRNA) are being processed, transported and cleaved. After all, miRNA becomes mature and functional.

1.2.1.2.1 MicroRNA genes

The primary transcripts of miRNA, which are called the primary-miRNA (pri-miRNA), can be hundreds to thousands of nucleotides long. They can be either monocistronic or polycistronic. They are 3' polyadenlylated, 5' "m^{7}Gppp" capped" and transcribed from miRNA genes by RNA polymerase II or III (Lee, Kim et al. 2004). Majority of the miRNA genes are regarded as independent transcribed units because they exist in the intergenic regions or in anti-sense directions to the flanking genes (Lee, Jeon et al. 2002; Lee, Kim et al. 2004; Lee and Kim 2007; Mraz, Dolezalova et al. 2012). Some miRNA genes are located in the host gene (intronic or exonic) and transcribed together while others have a clearly delineated transcription start site (TSS) and poly(A) tail (Rodriguez, Griffiths-Jones et al. 2004). Some miRNA genes such as miR-17-92 are even located in the introns of the genome and contain their own promoters (Ota, Tagawa et al. 2004). About 60% of miRNA genes lie on the intergenic region while others locate in the introns, exons or in combination with coding or non-coding genes (Rodriguez, Griffiths-Jones et al. 2004; Kim and Kim 2007). According to a study conducted in 2008, there was only 24 out of ~700 human exonic miRNAs (Maselli, Di Bernardo et al. 2008). Intronic miRNAs genes are usually located near the 5' end of the host gene (Zhou and

Lin 2008).

Up to 47% miRNA genes are usually clustered with multiple mature miRNA in zebrafish, mouse and human genomes (Lagos-Quintana, Rauhut et al. 2001; Griffiths-Jones, Saini et al. 2008; Thatcher, Bond et al. 2008). Most of them are evolutionarily conserved, suggesting miRNAs have important biological functions across different species (Pasquinelli, Reinhart et al. 2000).

1.2.1.2.2   MicroRNA processing

To synthesize mature miRNAs, the respective miRNA genes are firstly transcribed to pri-miRNAs. Except mirtons, the transcripts of the pri-miRNAs are cleaved by Drosha/Pasha (in animals) or Dicer-like 1 (DCL1) protein (in plants) to generate the precursor form, pre-miRNAs. Mirtrons, which are intron-encoded miRNAs, do not require the cleavage step as they will become pre-miRNAs after splicing (Okamura, Hagen et al. 2007; Zhu, Spriggs et al. 2008). In animals, the pri-miRNAs are transported out of the nucleus into the cytoplasm by a carrier protein exportin-5 and further processed into mature forms. Exportin-5 is a RanGTP-dependent pre-miRNA-specific export carrier protein. It transports dsRNA independently of their sequences (Bohnsack, Czaplinski et al. 2004). In plants, the pre-miRNAs are cleaved by DCL1 again into miRNA/miRNA* duplexes inside the nuclei. Then, the duplexes are transported out of the nuclei by an exportin-5 like protein, HASTY (HST), into the cytoplasm to form AGO silencing complexes (Kurihara and Watanabe 2004; Park, Wu et al. 2005).

Pre-miRNA is usually around 60-80 nt in size and folds into a stem-loop secondary structure. The mature miRNA can be found near the 5' or 3' end at the arm of the stem-loop. In animals, dicers cleave pre-miRNA into miRNA/miRNA* duplex, overhanging 2nt on the 3' end. The miRNA* is called the passenger strand or the star strand. The duplex is likely to be unwounded by RNA helicase A (Robb and Rana 2007) or Argonaute protein AGO2 (Diederichs and Haber 2007) into two separate strands. The star strand, which is complementary to the mature miRNA, is usually degraded. Because of the short-lived nature of the star strand, it is less abundant than the guide strand of the miRNA. In a recent research, however, some star stands are found to be as functional as the mature miRNAs (Okamura, Phillips et al. 2008). In addition, most plant miRNAs are 3' methylated, processed by HEN1, but this is not the case in animal miRNA (Axtell, Westholm et al. 2011). The single-stranded 21-24nt miRNA is then bound to the miRNA-induced silencing complex (miRISC) to exert its function (Lagos-Quintana, Rauhut et al. 2003; Lee, Ahn et al. 2003; Yi, Qin et al. 2003; Zhang, Kolb et al. 2004) (Figure 3)(Figure 4).

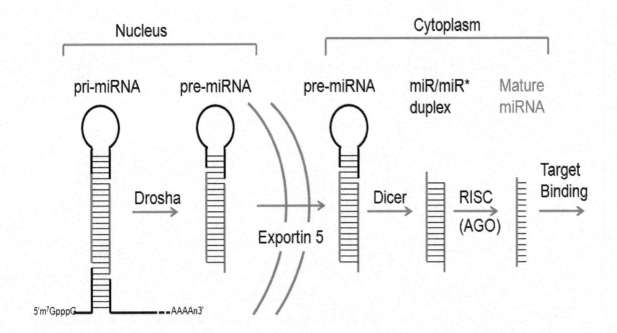

Figure 3. The miRNA biogenesis pathway in animals. Pri-miRNA is transcribed and cleaved by Drosha into pre-miRNA in the nuclus. The pre-miRNA is exported into cytoplasm by Exportin-5, and processed by Dicer protein into miR/miR* duplex. The duplex is then further processed by AGO protein into the RISC and is binded to the target.

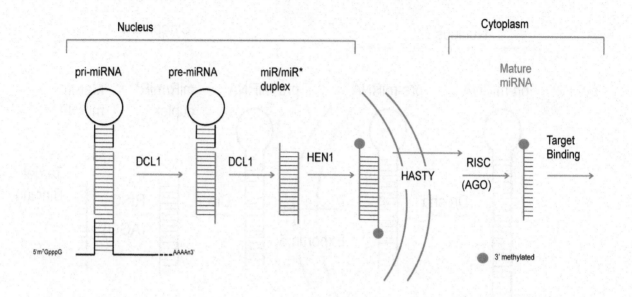

Figure 4. The miRNA biogenesis pathway in plants. Pri-miRNA is transcribed and cleaved by DCL1 into pre-miRNA then to miR/miR* duplex in the nuclus. HEN1 methylates the 3' end of the duplex and HASTY transported the duplex into the cytoplasm. The duplex is then further processed by AGO protein into the RISC and is binded to the target.

1.2.1.2.3 The miRNA-induced silencing complex (miRISC)

The miRNA-induced silencing complex (miRISC), which is a multiprotein complex, guides the mature miRNAs to target mRNAs. Argonaute proteins (AGO) form the core of miRISC and each AGO contains a dsRNA binding piwi-argonaute-zwille (PAZ) domain and a RNase H-like PIWI domain. There is a MID domain that usually lies between the PAZ and PIWI domains, having a basic pocket that binds with the Dicer-processed 5'-phosphate group of small RNA and anchors the small RNA on protein surface (Lee and Ambros 2001; Kiriakidou, Nelson et al. 2004; Brennecke, Stark et al. 2005; Aleman, Doench et al. 2007). The roles of AGO proteins are to bind with the single-stranded miRNA and maintain the miRISC conformation so as to benefit gene silencing functions. Besides, direct cleavage of the target mRNA (the silencing activity of AGO2) or recruitment of other silencing proteins to destabilize the targets is also achieved by AGO proteins. Different assistant proteins such as TRBP/PACT are also recruited by AGO to form the effective complex (Pratt and MacRae 2009).

1.2.1.2.4 miRNA-target recognition

In animals, the binding affinity between mRNA targets and miRNA is greatly enhanced by the seed region, a consecutive region with 7-nt or 6-nt long, of the miRNA. The seed region is located at the 5' 2-7nt or 2-8nt position of the miRNA (Brennecke, Stark et al. 2005; Brodersen and Voinnet 2009). In plants, most of the miRNA bound almost perfectly to the coding region of the target mRNA (Reinhart, Slack et al. 2000). The seed region matching sites on mRNA targets are highly conserved in human 3'-UTR regions (Lewis, Burge et al. 2005), with a significantly lower single nucleotide polymorphism (SNP) frequency than other conserved 3'-UTR regions, indicating there is a negative selection pressure on the seed binding sites (Chen and Rajewsky 2006).

In addition, researchers found that a mRNA target that is regulated by a specific miRNA in a particular cell type is not suppressed by the same miRNA in different cell types (Didiano and Hobert 2006). This indicated miRNA-target binding does not solely depend on the sequences complementary between the miRNA and mRNA, but is also influenced by other cell type specific factors, such as the RNA binding protein Dead-end 1 (Dnd1) was shown to block miRISC to 3'-UTR regions by binding itself to the U-rich 3'UTR sites (Kedde, Strasser et al. 2007).

1.2.1.3   Mechanism of actions

There are generally two factors mediating the functions of miRISC, Argonaute proteins and miRNAs. Argonaute proteins are further classified into 2 types: (I) slicer Argonaute that catalyze the cleavage of the target mRNA and (II) others Argonaute silencing complexes that repress translations or destabilize mRNAs. Silencing complex brings miRNA to its complementary mRNA in a perfectly complementary (usually plants) or imperfectly complementary manner (usually animals). At first, perfect complementary was thought to lead to site-specific cleavage and imperfectly complementary was thought to destabilize targets or inhibit translation. However, recent studies have proved that plant miRNAs also repress translation of their targets, although they are still near-perfect complementary to their target sequences (Brodersen, Sakvarelidze-Achard et al. 2008;

Lanet, Delannoy et al. 2009).

1.2.1.3.1   mRNA cleavage

In plants, miRNAs generally guide the cleavage of the complementary or nearly complementary mRNAs. Studies had shown that many miRNA targets were expressed at a higher level in RNAi protein mutant strains (e.g. HEN1, AGO1, HYL1) than the wild type. It indicated mutations in the RNAi proteins interrupted the miRNA-guided mRNA cleavage mechanisms, leading to accumulation of target mRNAs (Boutet, Vazquez et al. 2003; Vaucheret, Vazquez et al. 2004; Vazquez, Gasciolli et al. 2004). However, overexpression of miRNAs caused reduction in target mRNAs levels (Guo, Xie et al. 2005).

Arabidopsis encodes 10 AGO proteins. AGO4, AGO6 and AGO9 involve 24-nt small RNAs and responsible for transcriptional RNA silencing (Zilberman, Cao et al. 2003; Zheng, Zhu et al. 2007; Havecker, Wallbridge et al. 2010). AGO1 and AGO7 are slicer proteins that associated with 21-22nt small RNA (Baumberger and Baulcombe 2005; Qi, Denli et al. 2005; Montgomery, Howell et al. 2008). AGO1 and AGO10 are suggested to take part in translational repression, with an unknown pathway (Brodersen, Sakvarelidze-Achard et al. 2008; Mallory, Hinze et al. 2009).

Mammalian AGO2 (contains the RNaseH-like domain) is the only one out of the four Ago proteins in mammals that directly cleaves mRNA. Human AGO2 cleaves target mRNAs, which are highly complementary to the AGO2-miRNA complex. However, there are only few miRNAs that are perfectly complementary to mRNA targets in mammals (Liu, Carmell et al. 2004; Meister, Landthaler et al. 2004). Slicer cleavage of miRNA-targeted mRNA requires an A-form helix at the centre of the miRNA-mRNA duplex (Chiu and Rana 2003; Haley and Zamore 2004; Ma, Yuan et al. 2005). It is because there are usually mismatches and/or bulges on the centre of the animal miRNA-mRNA complex; therefore, direct mRNA decay is unlikely to be a widespread mechanism in mammals, but usually happens in the very-few mismatches miRNA-mRNA pairings in plants.

Some AGO proteins (e.g. human AGO1 and/or AGO2) and miRNA targets are localized in the cellular compartments called Processing bodies (P-bodies) (Liu, Valencia-Sanchez et al. 2005). P-bodies are cytoplasmic bodies that are used for degradation and storage of miRISC captured mRNAs. Inside the P-bodies, the mRNAs may be destabilized and/or repressed (Liu, Valencia-Sanchez et al. 2005; Sen and Blau 2005). Deletion of the P-bodies components such as Dcp1:Dcp2 complex, GW182 and Rck/p54, causes cessation of the repression to the target mRNAs *in vitro* (Jakymiw, Lian et al. 2005; Meister, Landthaler et al. 2005; Rehwinkel, Behm-Ansmant et al. 2005; Chu and Rana 2006). Some mRNAs that are sequestrated in P-bodies can exit the compartments and resume the translation process. Furthermore, some mRNAs can be deadenylated and degraded by decapping/Xrn1 pathway in the P-bodies. Deadenylase complex such as CCR4:NOT together with GW182 deadenylates and destabilizes mRNAs (Behm-Ansmant, Rehwinkel et al. 2006; Eulalio, Huntzinger et al. 2009). Then, decapping complex such as Dcp1:Dcp2 removes the m^7G cap of the mRNAs and degrades the mRNA by recruiting the 5' to 3' exoribonuclease, Xrn1p (Bagga, Bracht et al. 2005; Liu, Valencia-Sanchez et al. 2005; Rehwinkel, Behm-Ansmant et al. 2005; Behm-Ansmant, Rehwinkel et al. 2006). It is shown that about 60% of AGO1 targets are regulated by CAF1 and/or NOT1 in *Drosophila* (Eulalio, Huntzinger et al. 2009). However, the criteria for the miRISC complex to enter P-bodies are still unclear.

1.2.1.3.2 Translational repression

Translational inhibition happens when the degree of the decrease in protein product is greater than the degree of decrease in mRNA level. However, the mechanisms for translational inhibition are still not fully understood at this moment. Different mechanisms and models with contradictory results were reported for miRNA-guided translational repression. These proposed mechanisms involve different steps in the translation processes. However, in general, there are three main processes involved in translation: ribosome initiation, elongation and termination.

In the early 1990s, studies on *C. elegans* demonstrated that the lin-4 miRNA repressed lin-14 gene expression by binding to 3'-UTR of the lin-14 mRNA (Arasu, Wightman et al. 1991; Lee, Feinbaum et al. 1993; Wightman, Ha et al. 1993). Lin-4 was thought to repress protein translation instead of destabilizing the mRNA because the levels of lin-14 mRNA and its poly(A)-tail length were not affected by lin-4 (Olsen and Ambros 1999). The lin-4 did not alter the polyribosomes association with the lin-14 mRNA. This indicated lin-4 did not inhibit translation in the initiation step but at the later elongation or termination step.

Studies on *C.elegans* and plants suggested miRNAs and their mRNA targets co-sediment with polyribosomes. MiRNAs inhibited protein translation because of the rapid "ribosome drop-off" from target mRNA during the elongation or termination steps (Seggerson, Tang et al. 2002; Petersen, Bordeleau et al. 2006; Lanet, Delannoy et al. 2009) . Peptides were synthesized immaturely due to the "ribosome drop-off" from the translating mRNAs. However, the suggested immature polypeptides chains cannot be detected by antibodies so far. This phenomenon proposed miRISC may recruit protease that would degrade the nascent polypeptides chains immediately. Another possibility was the nascent polypeptides were indeed not being synthesized due to the blocking in translation initiation (Nottrott, Simard et al. 2006).

Evidence of miRNA-guided repression at post-initiation ribosome entry step were reported from two studies. The inhibition of miRNAs translation was mediated by cap-dependent and/or cap-independent, which involved the internal ribosome entry site (IRES) (Petersen, Bordeleau et al. 2006; Lytle, Yario et al. 2007). Since IRES-mediated and cap-dependent initiated translations are of two different mechanisms, it is still unknown whether miRNAs inhibit translation initiation in miRNA specific manner or involve both mechanisms.

Other studies suggested that miRNAs interfered with cap-dependent translation initiation. Non-functional ApppG caps in reporter mRNAs were resistant to inhibition *in vitro*, while those mRNAs with m^7G caps were repressed a thousand folds more. Furthermore, the degree of miRNA inhibition was increased by adding an excess amount of eIF4F complex *in vitro*. These data supported the miRNA-guided translation inhibited translation at cap-dependent initiation steps (Humphreys, Westman et al. 2005; Mathonnet, Fabian et al. 2007; Thermann and Hentze 2007). Indeed, in some studies, IRES-mediated initiation was resistant to miRNA-guided repression (Humphreys, Westman et al. 2005; Pillai, Bhattacharyya et al. 2005). An explanation for the above observations was that miRNA-loaded AGO2 (in human) may compete with the eIF4 complex for the binding of 5' m^7G cap. It was supported by human AGO2 that contained a m^7G cap binding motif (Kiriakidou, Tan et al. 2007). In a *Drosophila* cells study, it was found that interaction between the cap-binding motif of AGO2 and GW182 was existed (Eulalio, Huntzinger et al. 2008). GW182 was an Ago interacting protein that was required for miRNA-guided translational repression (Rehwinkel, Behm-Ansmant et al. 2005). It was possible that the lost of competing ability with eIF4 for binding 5' capped structure in AGO2 complex was due to the inability to recruit GW182.

Different models for miRNA-guided translation repression involved different translation steps. It is unclear that whether the arguments are due to different experimental approaches or whether miRNA mechanisms for translational repression is miRNA and/or targets specific. More research have to be done in the future to reveal the whole picture.

1.2.1.4 Roles of microRNA

Thousands of miRNAs have been identified after the discovery of miRNAs. The latest release of the miRBase, the miRNA database online, miRBase release 19.0 (miRBase 2012), included 25,141 miRNAs in 193 different species of animals, plants, viruses and unicellular organisms (mirbase 2012). MicroRNAs involve many biological pathways in eukaryotes. Knockout and/or knockdown RNAi proteins as well as particular miRNAs are valuable experiments to study the functions of miRNA inside the organisms. In animals, *Canorhabditis elegans*, *Drosophila melanogaster*, *Mus musculus* and *Homo sapiens* are the main models to conduct *in vitro* and/or *in vivo* miRNA functional studies. MiRNAs in animals are involved in:

1)   Cell differentiation and development: The let7 miRNA can stabilize the self-renewing verse differentiated cell fates in mouse embryonic stem cells (Melton, Judson et al. 2010). The let-7 in *C. elegans* regulates the developmental transition between the last larval stage (L4) and the adult stage (Reinhart, Slack et al. 2000; Slack, Basson et al. 2000).

2)   Viral infection: miRNAs regulate genes that involve in innate immunity and defense RNA and DNA viruses in host cell (O'Connell, Taganov et al. 2007; O'Hara, Mott et al. 2009). Expression of miR-122 works through IFN-ß and inhibits replication of hepatitis C virus (HCV) (Lanford, Hildebrandt-Eriksen et al. 2010).

3)   Immunity: miR-223 regulates the differentiation and activation of granulocytes and the inflammatory response. Loss of miR-223 results in a cell-autonomous increase in the granulocyte progenitor's number and an expanded granulocytic compartment. Those granulocytes are hypermature and hypersensitive to stimulations and show an increment of fungicidal activity in mice (Johnnidis, Harris et al. 2008). A report in 2012 stated that 68% of known immune-related pre-miRNAs were present in the human breast milk exosome. These miRNAs were more resistant to harsh conditions than the normal one. It

was possible that miRNAs from mother's breast milk exosomes played an important role in infant immune system (Zhou, Li et al. 2012).

4)   Cancer: The miRNA profiles of cancer patients are usually different from the normal individuals. A microchip study profiled human and mouse miRNA expression. It discovered each breast cancer tissue had specific patterns of miRNA profile (Liu, Calin et al. 2004). In addition, the blood level of miR-15 and miR-16 in 68% chronic lymphocytic leukemia patients were found to be absent or down-regulated (Calin, Dumitru et al. 2002). The let-7 miRNA family was shown to inhibit the proto-oncogene, RAS protein, expression in human cancer cell lines (Johnson, Grosshans et al. 2005; Sassen, Miska et al. 2008). Loss or reduction in let-7 showed an upregulation of RAS protein, promoting the growth of cancer cells in lung. The poor prognosis of lung cancer was also found to correlate with the reduction of let-7 expression (Takamizawa, Konishi et al. 2004).

5)   Cardiac diseases: Inhibition of miR-133 increases cardiac hypertrophy *in vivo*. Muscle specific miR-133a-1 and miR-133a-2 are related to muscle development. Lacking both of them results in lethal ventricular septal defects (VSD) in about 50% of double-mutant embryos or neonates (Liu, Bezprozvannaya et al. 2008).

6)   Signal Transmission: Exosomes are membrane vesicles that are released into the extracellular environment. Exosomes promote communication between cells. MiRNAs are found in exosomes, and can be functional in the destination cells once they are transported by exosomes (Valadi, Ekstrom et al. 2007).

In plants, *Arabidopsis thaliana* and rice (*Oryza sativa*) are the most common models in miRNAs studies. MiRNAs in plants are involved in:

43

1)   Organ development: A) Leaf morphogenesis: miR-JAW regulates leaf and other organ development by targeting TCP genes. Overexpression of miR-JAW downregulates five TCP genes, causing epinasty of the cotyledon, fruit abnormalities, secretion of leaf margins and delay in flowering (Palatnik, Allen et al. 2003). B) Identity of floral organs and flowering time: miR-156 targets SPL transcription factors. Overexpression of miR-156 causes late flowering in *A. thaliana*. Besides, miR-172 targets AP2 gene. Overexpression of miR-172 results in lacking AP2 gene, leading to the replacement of perianth organs by reproductive organs (Jack 2004). C) Auxin homeostasis and root development: Auxin signaling pathway plays critical roles in plant growth and development. Many genes in the pathway are targeted by miRNAs. For example, miR-160 targets ARF10, ARF16 and ARF17 (Rhoades, Reinhart et al. 2002). In a study, ARF17 expression was increased by introducing miRNA-resistant-ARF17. This resulted in pleiotropic developmental abnormalities, such as root growth defects (Mallory, Bartel et al. 2005).

2)   Feedback regulation in small RNA pathway: Dicer-like 1 (DCL1) expression level can be feedback regulated by miR-162 (Xie, Kasschau et al. 2003). Whereas AGO1 is targeted by miR168. Overexpressing miR168-resistant AGO1 affects miRNA pathway. The phenotypes of plants were similar to the mutants of *dcl1* (Vaucheret, Vazquez et al. 2004). AGO2 also includes a binding site for miR403 in its 3' UTR region (Allen, Xie et al. 2005).

1.2.1.5   MicroRNAs in fungi

RNAi proteins such as Dicer and Argonaute have been identified in many fungi, such as the fungal model strains: the filamentous fungus *Neurospora crassa* (Fulci and Macino 2007) and the fission yeast *Schizosaccharomyces pombe* (Sigova, Rhind et al. 2004). Although RNAi proteins were lost in the famous budding yeast *Saccharomyces cerevisiae*, its closely related species *Saccharomyces castelli* encoded a defected but functional Dicer-like homolog (Figure 5).

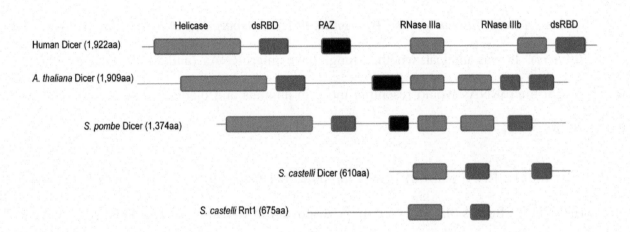

Figure 5. Dicers' helicase domains, double stranded RNA binding domains (dsRBD), PAZ domains, RNase III domain in different organisms. Dicer and the dicer-like protein, Rnt1, in *S. castelli* have only one RNase III domain and lack PAZ and helicase domain.

Large numbers of novel miRNAs have been identified in animals, plants, insects, algae and slime mould after the establishment on the field of microRNA since 2001. Fungi were targets for the identification of miRNAs. However, even in 2005, there was no endogenous microRNAs have yet been reported in fungi but only some antisense transcripts that had been found in the genome of *Cryptococcus neoformans* (Loftus, Fung et al. 2005). No plant or animal-like microRNAs was found in *Aspergillus* species by computational analysis of six *Aspergillus* genomes (*Aspergillus nidulans*, *Aspergillus oryzae*, *Aspergillus fumigatus*, *Aspergillus terreus*, *Aspergillus clavatus*, and *Neosartorya fischeri*). It was unclear whether fungi have microRNAs, and, if they have, whether fungal microRNAs would resemble those in animals and plants. (McGuire and Galagan 2008).

The RNAi pathway of *N. crassa* has been studied extensively; it is the model in filamentous fungus that involved in the discovery of fungal Dicer-regulated siRNA events: quelling and meiotic silencing of unpaired DNA (MSUD). The two Dicer-like proteins in *N. crassa* were found to be redundant in cleaving dsRNA into siRNA (Catalanotto, Pallotta et al. 2004). The Dicer-like proteins in *N. crassa* was also responsible for the production of qiRNA, a novel class of small interfering RNA (~21nt). Endogenous dsRNA, which originated from rDNA loci, was produced when DNA damage had been induced by the treatment of DNA-damaging agents. The qiRNA was associated with QDE-2 (Argonaute-like protein). It was suggested that qiRNAs responded to DNA damage by inhibiting protein synthesis (Lee, Chang et al. 2009).

In 2010, miRNA-like RNAs (milRNAs) were identified in *N.crassa* by Lee and his research group (Lee, Li et al. 2010). At least 25 milRNAs were identified by analyzing the deep sequencing reads of QDE-2-associated small RNAs. These milRNAs were similar to classical miRNAs: 1) they were predominantly originated from one strand of hairpin-like single-stranded RNA precursors; 2) they had strong preference for U at the 5' ends; 3) they repressed genes expression; 4) their predicted mRNA targets expression levels increased in RNAi proteins mutants. However, milRNAs of *N. crassa* were found to have diverse pathway for biogenesis. The biogenesis required different combinations of Dicer, QDE-2, QIP, MRPL3 and others. At least four milRNAs production pathways were identified:

1)   *milR-1* milRNAs required Dicer to cleave primary *milR-1* into pre-*milR-1*, then bound to Argonaute QDE-2 and together with QIP. Pre-*milR-1* was processed into mature *milR-1*.

2)   *milR-2* was produced independently with Dicer. QDE-2 bound to pre-*milR-2* and cleaved the star milRNA for further processing.

3)   *milR-3* production followed the canonical plant miRNA pathway. Dicer was the only catalytic enzyme in the maturation.

4)   *milR-4* maturation required MRPL3 but only partially dependent on Dicer.

This was the first study to identify functional fungal miRNAs (Lee, Li et al. 2010) (Figure 6). However, no biological role of milRNAs has been determined as there was no phenotypic difference among the knockout mutants.

Zhou and his groups had identified milRNAs in another fungus, a plant pathogenic fungus *Sclerotinia sclerotiorum*, in 2012 (Zhou, Fu et al. 2012). *S. sclerotiorum* is classified in the phylum of Ascomycota and causes white mould in plants. Analysis of the deep sequencing results had revealed 2 milRNAs and 42 milRNAs candidates. *SS-milR-1* and *SS-milR-C2* showed differential expression in different developmental process of *S. sclerotiorum*. *SS-milR-1* level was reduced in sclerotial development. *SS-milR-C2* expression levels remained the same at different time points. In this study, milRNAs candidates were predicted and two of them were confirmed by Northern Blotting (Zhou, Fu et al. 2012). Another group also identified milRNAs in the entopathogenic fungi *Metarhizium anisopliae*. They predicted 15 milRNAs from the fungus and found that there is differential expression of the milRNAs in mycelium and conidiogenssis stage (Zhou, Wang et al. 2012). However, no mRNA targets of the two *S. sclerotiorum* milRNAs have been predicted. Also, no RNAi protein mutants have been created in the two fungi. The maturation process of these milRNAs in *S.sclerotiorum* and *M. anisopliae* remains uncertain. Although the differential expression of milRNAs may indicate they have important biological roles (such as development and conidiogenesis), it needs further study to confirm.

In 2013, a group discovered miRNAs in the human pathogenic fungus *C. neoformans*, they found that the miRNAs caused transgene silencing via the canonical RNAi pathway. The identified miRNAs predicted targets are mostly against transposable elements (TEs) and pseudogenes (Jiang, Yang et al. 2012).

N. crassa and *M. anisopliae* do not contain potential homologues of the Drosha and Pasha proteins, that may produce pre-miRNAs from pri-miRNAs as those in animals, suggesting the difference between the biogenesis in milRNAs (four pathways of milRNAs in the fungi, *N. crassa*) and miRNAs (in animals) (Zhou, Wang et al. 2012).

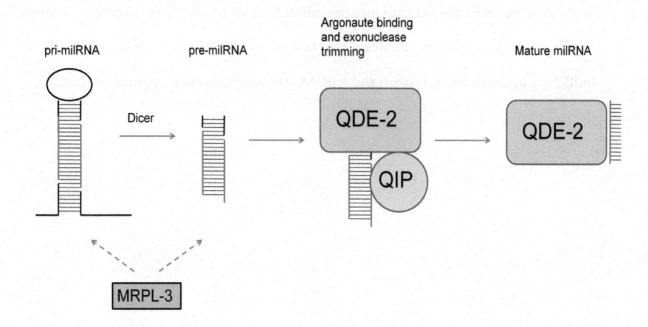

Figure 6. Schematic diagram of the milRNAs mechanisms in *N.crassa* (Lee, Li et al. 2010). Pri-milRNA is dicer dependent and MRPL-3 has roles in the maturation of pri-milRNA or pre-milRNA. The pre-milRNA is further processed by QDE-2 and QIP into mature milRNA. The mature milRNA binds to QDE-2 to exert its gene targeting activities.

1.3   Rationale and scope of present study

MicroRNAs (miRNAs) are small non-coding endogenous RNAs of about 21-22nt in average. They play important roles in post-transcriptional gene regulation in animals and plants (Bartel 2004). With the advent of molecular and bioinformatics tools, numerous miRNAs have been identified in animals, plants, virus and unicellular organisms, with more than 25,000 miRNAs being included in the miRNA database, miRBase release 19.0 (Griffiths-Jones, Grocock et al. 2006). Although small RNA pathways have been found in various fungi, the existence of miRNAs and their roles were less well understood. Recently, milRNAs have been identified in *N. crassa, S. sclerotiorum, M. anisopliae* and *C. neoformans* (Lee, Li et al. 2010; Jiang, Yang et al. 2012; Zhou, Fu et al. 2012; Zhou, Wang et al. 2012). MilRNAs did not show essential features in dicers knockout mutants of *N.crassa* and *C. neoformans* whereas dicers knockout mutants in animals and/or plants greatly influenced the growth and their development in certain organisms. However, their regulatory functions and pathways, potential roles in virulence and the involvement in fungal dimorphism of milRNAs were largely unknown.

P. marneffei is the most important thermal dimorphic pathogenic fungus which infects over 10% of HIV-positive patients in Southeast Asia. Therefore, it is valuable to investigate whether miRNAs exist in *P. marneffei* and their potential roles. It is hypothesized that miRNAs exist in *P. marnaffei* and involve in virulence and dimorphism. This study was carried out to test these hypotheses. In the first part of the study, two dicers-like and argonaute-like QDE-2 proteins were identified in *P. marneffei* genome and their knockout mutants were created. Their contributions to virulence were examined in macrophage cell lines and mice challenging model. The contributions of dicer-like and argonaute-like proteins in hydrogen peroxide susceptibility and dimorphic switch were also examined. In the second part of the study, based on the available genome sequence data, milRNAs were identified in *P. marneffei* in both mycelial and yeast phase using high-throughput sequencing technology. Sequence analysis revealed 24 potential milRNA candidates, which were more abundantly expressed in mycelial than yeast phase of *P. marneffei*. Northern blot analysis confirmed the expression of two milRNAs, *PM-mil-M1* and *PM-milR-M2*, which were dependent on a Dicer-like protein. The milRNAs targets were also predicted. These findings provided the first evidence for the existence of milRNA in human fungal pathogens, demonstrated differential expression of milRNA during different phases in thermally dimorphic fungi, and suggested the argonaute-like QDE-2 protein is involved in virulence in mice model.

CHAPTER 2 MATERIALS AND METHODS

2.1 *P. marneffei* strains and growth conditions

P. marneffei strain PM1 was isolated from a HIV-negative penicilliosis patient in Hong Kong. Knock-out mutant strains were generated as described in later section. *P. marneffei* was grown on Sabouraud dextrose agar (SDA) (Oxoid, Cambridge, UK) at 37°C for 10 days for yeast cultures or at room temperature for 7 days for mould cultures for the collection of conidia. Conidia and yeast cells were collected by scraping and resuspension in PBS with 0.1% Tween-20 followed by two washes in sterile PBS. Liquid cultures of *P. marneffei* for nucleic acid extraction were grown in BHI medium (Difco, NJ, USA) in a shaker at 37°C for yeast or at room temperature for mould for 48 -72 hours. Conidia and yeast cells were counted using a hemocytometer.

2.2 DNA Extraction for PCR Amplification

DNA extraction of *P. marneffei* for PCR amplification of the flanking regions of *dcl-1*, *dcl-2* and *qde-2* for constructing gene knockout plasmids was performed using the MasterPure Yeast DNA Purification kit (Epicentre, Wisconsin, USA) according to manufacturer's manual. Yeast cells of *P. marneffei* were harvested in 300μl Yeast Cell Lysis Solution. One microliter of RNase A solution were then added to lysates and mixed using vortex for about 30 seconds. Cells were then incubated at 65°C water bath for 15 minutes with gentle agitation. Cell lysates were then placed on ice for at least five minutes before adding 150 μl of MPC Protein Precipitation Reagent. Cell lysates were

53

followed by vortex mix for 30 seconds. Cell debris was then centrifuged in a bench microcentrifuge for 10 minutes at 13,000 rpm. Supernatants were transferred to microcentrifuge tubes with 500 µl of isopropanol each. Samples were then mixed by inversion. DNA was pelleted in each tube by centrifugation for 10 minutes at ≥13,000 rpm. Supernatant were then discarded and pellets were washed with 500µl of 70% ethanol. Traces of ethanol solutions were removed by centrifugation and pipetting. DNA pellets were allowed to air dry for 10 minutes. DNA pellets were dissolved in 35 µl of TE Buffer and incubated at 45-50°C for 30 minutes. DNA samples were then stored at -20°C.

2.3 PCR amplification and sequencing

PCR amplification for constructing the *dcl-1*,*dcl-2* and *qde-2* knockout plasmids were performed using iProof High-Fidelity DNA Polymerase (Bio-Rad, California, USA). PCR amplification for screening of *dcl-1*, *dcl-2* and *qde-2* knockout mutants were performed using AmpliTaq Gold® DNA Polymerase (Applied Biosystems, Inc., California, USA) according to manufacturer's instructions. The PCR conditions were as followed: DNA were amplified for 32 cycles at denaturation step for 94°C (1 minute), annealing step for 5°C above the melting temperature of respective primers for 30secs and extension step for 72°C, 1 min/kb bps. Thermal cycling steps were performed using an ABI GeneAmp® 9700 60-Well PCR System. Visualization of DNA samples were achieved by agarose gel electrophoresis using 1.5% SeaKem® LE Agarose gel (Lonza Rockland, Inc., Maine, USA) in Tris/Boric Acid/EDTA (TBE) buffer (Bio-Rad, California, USA) with Lambda DNA/Eco47I (AvaII) Marker, 13 as the size marker and a 6X DNA Loading Dye (Thermo Fisher Scientific, Massachusetts, USA). Gels were stained in 0.5 µl/ml ethidium bromide solution (Bio-Rad, California, USA) for 15 minutes, rinsed with fresh TBE buffer and photographed under ultraviolet illumination using a Gel Doc™ XR+ System (Bio-Rad, California, USA).

DNA sequencing procedures were as follow: PCR products were purified using QIAquick PCR Purification Kit (Qiagen, Hilden, Germany) or QIAquick Gel Extraction Kit (Qiagen, Hilden, Germany) according to manufacturer's instructions. Both strands of PCR products were sequenced with respective forward and reverse primers using a ABI PRISM® 3700 Genetic Analyzer (Applied Biosystems, Inc., California, USA).

2.4   Total RNA extraction and reverse transcription

Total RNA extraction for reverse transcription of *dcl-1*, *dcl-2*, *qde-2* mRNA for RT-PCR and real-time qPCR was performed using the Ambion RiboPure-Yeast kit (Applied Biosystems, Inc., California, USA) according to manufacturer's protocols. Mycelia or yeast cells of *P. marneffei* from BHI culture were harvested in 480µl lysis buffer, 48µl 10% SDS and 480µl Phenol:Chloroform:IAA. The samples were then disrupted with Zirconia beads using TissueLyser II (Qiagen, Hilden, Germany) at top speed for two minutes twice with 30 seconds resting interval. Disrupted samples were centrifuged for five minutes at room temp. The upper aqueous phase was transferred to a fresh 50 ml tube. Binding Buffer of 2ml and 100% ethanol of 1.25ml were added. The mixtures were then passed through the Filter Cartridge and centrifuged for 15-30secs at 13,000 rpm 700µl each time until the entire sample was filtered. Flow-through was discarded. The filter was washed with 700 µl Wash Solution 1 (Applied Biosystems, Inc., California, USA) by centrifuging for 15-30secs at 13,000 rpm. The filter was washed twice with 500 µl Wash Solution 2/3 (Applied Biosystems, Inc., California, USA) by same centrifuging time and speed. The Filter Cartridge was centrifuged for 1 minute at 13,000 rpm to remove excess solutions on the filter and allowed to air dry for 2 mins. Finally, RNA was eluted twice using 95°C preheated 50 µl Elution Solution.

DNase I treatment was performed to remove contaminating chromosomal DNA according to instructions in the RiboPure-Yeast kit. 10 µl 10X DNase 1 Buffer and 4 µl DNase I was added to each 100µl RNA samples. The mixture was incubated at 37°C for at least 30 mins. Then 11 µL DNase Inactivation Reagent was added to the mixture. The mixture was mixed using vortex for 15 secs and incubated at room temperature for 5 mins. After 5 min, DNase Inactivation Reagent was pelleted by centrifugation at 13,000 rpm for 3 minutes and the supernatant containing RNA was transferred to a fresh tube and stored at –80°C before use.

Reverse transcription of the total RNA was performed using the SuperScript III reverse transcription kit (Invitrogen, California, USA) according to manufacturer's instructions with oligo d(T) primer. Thermal cycling steps were performed using an ABI GeneAmp® 9700 60-Well PCR System (Applied Biosystems, Inc., California, USA).

2.5 Identification and characterization of DCL-1, DC2 and QDE-2 in *P. marneffei*

2.5.1 Gene annotation

Based on the predicted protein sequences of corresponding genes from *N. crassa* (DCL-1 Accession: Q7S8J7.1, DCL-2 Accession: Q7SCC1.3, QDE-2 GenBank: ABQ45366.1), putative *dcl-1*, *dcl-2* and *qde-2* genes in *P. marneffei* strain PM1 draft genome sequence were searched using BLASTP algorithm. Introns were predicted by performing pairwise alignment with the annotated *Talaromyces stipitatus* (teleomorph of *Penicillium emmonsii*) and *P. marneffei* strain ATCC 18224 genome sequences. The complete coding sequences of *dcl-1*, *dcl-2* and *qde-2* of *P. marneffei* were PCR amplified from cDNA using primers designed based on *P. marneffei* genome sequence data as described previously with modifications (Table 1) (Woo, Tam et al. 2010).

2.5.2 Phylogenic analysis

To perform phylogenetic analysis, putative *dcl-1*, *dcl-2* and *qde-2* homologues from representative fungal species were retrieved using BLASTP against the GenBank database. Nucleotide sequences of the internal transcribed spacer (ITS) regions were obtained from GenBank. Phylogenetic trees were constructed using the maximum-likelihood method with 1000 bootstrap replicates with Mega 5.1 (MM). WAG+F+G (for *dcl-1* and *dcl-2*) and rtREV+G (for *qde-2*) amino acid substitution models, K2+G nucleotides substitution models (for ITS) with 5 gamma categories were used. Nine-hundred and fourteen, 764 and 525 amino acid positions of *dcl-1*, *dcl-2* and *qde-2* respectively, and 465 nucleotides positions of ITS, were used for analysis. Domains were predicted using the Conserved Domains Database of NCBI and PFAM (http://pfam.sanger.ac.uk/search?tab=searchSequenceBlock) and manual inspection of multiple alignments with homologous sequences.

2.6   Plasmids construction

2.6.1   Generation of $dcl-1^{KO}$, $dcl-2^{KO}$, $qde-2^{KO}$, dcl^{DKO} deletion mutant of *P. marneffei*

The deletion mutants were generated by homologous recombination (Fig. 7). Based on *dcl-1*, *dcl-2* and *qde-2* gene sequences from *P. marneffei* strain PM1, primers were designed to amplify upstream and downstream fragments of *dcl-1, dcl-2* and *qde-2* for the construction of the corresponding knockout constructs using the vector pAN7-1 (Punt, Oliver et al. 1987). The flanking sequences upstream and downstream of *dcl-1, dcl-2* and *qde-2* were amplified by PCR using DNA extracted from strain PM1 and primers shown in Table 1. PCR products of upstream and downstream flanking fragments were ligated into corresponding restriction sites of plasmid pAN7-1 to generate the knock-out plasmids pAN7-*dcl-1* (PW1634), pAN7-*dcl-2* (PW1633) and pAN7-*qde-2* (PW1665) as shown in Fig. 7. The resultant plasmids were linearized with *Ahd*I and transformed to strain PM1 according to previous publications (Sanglard, Ischer et al. 1996). SDA supplemented with 150 µg/ml hygromycin B was used as selection medium. To construct dcl^{DKO}, PCR products of *dcl-1* flanking fragments were ligated into vector pAN8-1 (Punt, Oliver et al. 1987) as described previously (Mattern, Punt et al. 1988) to generate the knock-out plasmid pAN8-*dcl-1* (Fig. 7). pAN8-*dcl-1* (PW1635) was linearized with *Ahd*I and transformed to $dcl-2^{KO}$ to generate the double mutant dcl^{DKO}, using SDA supplemented with 100 µg/ml phleomycin as selection medium.

Table 1. Primers used in this study

Gene Targets	Primers	Purpose
Upstream of	PW10929 5'-GAAGATCTCCGTAGTGCTTCTGATTGGTCTGAG-3'	pAN7-1 cloning
dcl-1	PW10930 5'-GAAGATCTTCTTTTGCGGCCTTTGTAAGTCTG-3'	(*Bgl*II and
Downstream of	PW10931 5'-TGATTGAAGATCCTCCCAAGGTTG-3'	*Hind*III)
dcl-1	PW10932 5'-CCCAAGCTTGGGTGGTTCGTGAGATAGGTGGTGGATA -3'	
Upstream of	PW13339 5'-GAAGATCTCGCCGAACAAACGGAAGAAGGAGA-3'	pAN7-1 cloning
dcl-2	PW13340 5'-TGGCTTCTCCGAAGCTCTCTATGG-3'	(*Bgl*II and *Sfo*I)
Downstream of	PW13341 5'-ATAGGCGCCCCTAGTCGATTTTCATGAACGGACC-3'	
dcl-2	PW13342 5'-ATAGGCGCCGGATTACATAACATACCGTCGGCTG-3'	
Upstream of	PW12475 5'-ACCCAATAAGGATGAGGAAGTTCGG-3'	pAN7-1 cloning
qde-2	PW12476 5'-GAAGATCT AAGTCAGTCGCAATCTCGTCCCG-3'	(*Bgl*II and *Sbf*I)
Downstream of	PW12718 5'-GACCTGCAGGACACATCACCAAGTGAAGTGTCAC-3'	
qde-2	PW12719 5'-GACCTGCAGGATCCGCTTGACTCCAGGTGGTA -3'	
Upstream of	PW10929 5'-GAAGATCTCCGTAGTGCTTCTGATTGGTCTGAG-3'	pAN8-1 cloning
dcl-1	PW10930 5'-GAAGATCTTCTTTTGCGGCCTTTGTAAGTCTG-3'	(*Bgl*II and *Sfo*I)
Downstream of	PW12799 5'-ATAGGCGCCTGATTGAAGATCCTCCCAAGGTTG-3'	
dcl-1	PW12800 5'-ATAGGCGCCTGGTTCGTGAGATAGGTGGTGGATA -3'	
dcl-1	PW13343 5'-TTTACGGGACGTAAATGGCGGCCTA-3'	qPCR
	PW13344 5'-AATTCTAGGCGCTGGTAAGTCGGC-3'	
	PW21945 5'-ATGTTGGAGACTCTTACCCTGG-3'	cDNA
	PW22072 5'-CTCGGCATTCCATAGTTTGT-3'	amplification &
	PW22073 5'-GCCGAGGTTTCATGGAAAGA-3'	sequencing
	PW22074 5'-CGGTTCAGCTGGAGAAAACA-3'	
	PW22075 5'-CGTCAAACCTTCATTCTGGA-3'	
	PW22076 5'-CGGTGTTGAATAAATTCCTG-3'	
	PW22077 5'-ATATCTTTATTCGTTGGAAGTCCG-3'	

	PW21946 5'-TACATCACGGGACTCGGGGA-3'	
	PW21943 5'-ATGGCCATAGAGAGCTTCGG-3'	
	PW22066 5'-TCGGCCAAAACGTCCCTTTG-3'	
	PW22067 5'-CTCATCTCTTGAGCGTGCAC-3'	
dcl-2	PW13347 5'-GTGTGAAGTGATATTGCCAAAGGG-3'	qPCR
	PW13348 5'-CATTTGTAACGGTTCAGCTGGAG-3'	
	PW22068 5'-CGATGATGAATGGTCGTGAA-3'	cDNA
	PW22069 5'-GATGCAAAATCTTGGAATGG-3'	amplification &
	PW22070 5'-GCATCAGGTGCATTTCTTGG-3'	sequencing
	PW22071 5'-CGATTCCTTGCTAGACCACTTCG-3'	
	PW21944 5'-CACTGCCGGCTTGACTGTCC-3'	
	PW21947 5'-ATGTCCAGCGGGTATAGACG-3'	
	PW22078 5'-TCTAGCCGAGCCTTGCCCTT-3'	
	PW22079 5'-CTAGTACAGCCTCGGTAGACA-3'	
	PW22080 5'-ACCTTCAGAGACTCCATCGC-3'	
qde-2	PW14804 5'-GCCTCATCAAAATCCCCGGT-3'	qPCR
	PW14805 5'-GGAGAAACGACGACACCCAT-3'	
	PW22081 5'-CCGCCCTTCCTGAGAACATT-3'	cDNA
	PW22082 5'-TTAGATATAGAACATCGTGT-3'	amplification &
		sequencing
actin	PW20631 5'-GAACGTGAAATCGTCCGT-3'	qPCR
	PW20160 5'-AGCAAGAATGGAACCACC-3'	

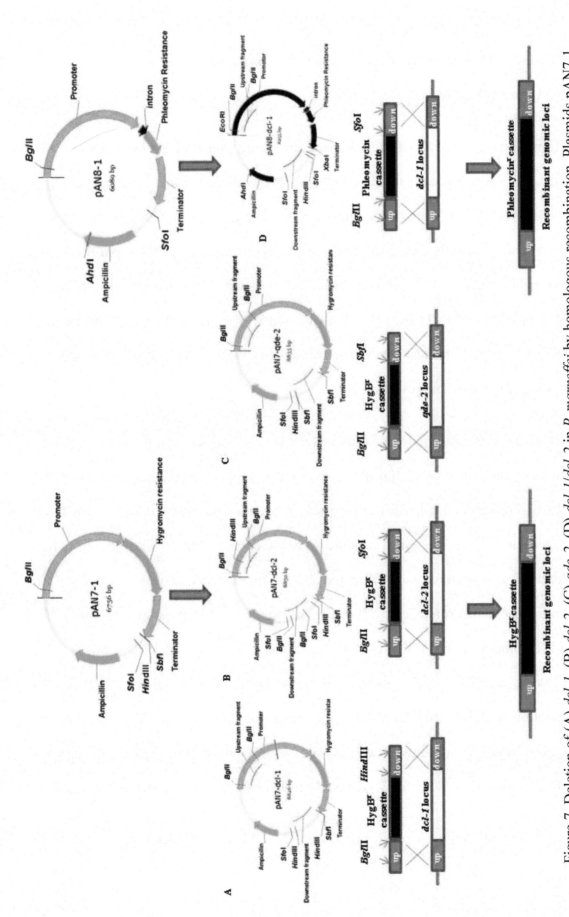

Figure 7. Deletion of (A) *dcl-1*, (B) *dcl-2*, (C) *qde-2*, (D) *dcl-1/dcl-2* in *P. marneffei* by homologous recombination. Plasmids pAN7-1 and pAN8-1 were used to construct the knockout plasmids of pAN7-*dcl-1*, pAN7-*dcl-2*, pAN7-*qde-2* and pAN8-*dcl-1* respectively.

2.7   Fungal transformation and screening for mutants

2.7.1   Transformation of *P. marneffei*

Competent cells of *P. marneffei* yeast form were prepared for transformation by inoculating in Yeast Peptone Dextrose (YPD) broth (Sigma-Aldrich, Missouri, USA) at a cell density of 10^8/ml. Then the broth was incubated at 37°C with shaking at 250 rpm for 24 hrs. The yeast cells were then harvested by centrifugation at 2500 rpm for 5 min. Supernatant was discarded. The cell pellet was washed with cold 25 ml TE buffer (10mM Tris-HCl, 1mM EDTA, pH 7.5) twice and with cold 5 ml Li-TE buffer (0.1M lithium acetate in TE buffer) once. The yeast cells were then resuspended in equal volume of Li-TE buffer and rested on ice.

Heat shock transformation of *P. marneffei* was performed as follow: To each fifty microliters of competent cells, 300 µl polyethylene glycol (PEG) (sigma-Aldrich) buffer (40% PEG 4000 in Li-TE buffer), 10 µg single stranded sheared salmon sperm DNA (Invitrogen) and 1.5 µg linearized plasmid were added sequentially with mixing before each addition. The mixtures were incubated at 30°C for 30 min and heat-shocked at 42°C for 40 min. The transformed yeast cells were collected by short spins up to 8,000rpm for three to four times. The yeast cells were then inoculated to 10 ml YPD broth at 37°C with shaking at 250 rpm for 24 h. The transformed yeast cells were pelleted by centrifugation at 2,500 rpm for 5 min and plated on hygromycin B (80 µg/ml) for pAN7-1 or phleomycin (100ug/ml) for pAN8-1 selective SDA plates (75 ml). The plates were then incubated at 37°C for 2 weeks. Then hygromycin B or phleomycin resistant colonies were picked to new selective plates and further confirmation of knockout mutants.

2.7.2   Confirmation of knockout mutants

To screen for knockout mutants of *dcl-1*, *dcl-2* and *qde-2*, the transformed clones of *P. marneffei* were screened and confirmed by PCR using three sets of primers. For screening the clones of pAN7-*dcl-2*, a 1275 bp and a 1547 bp fragments would be amplified LPW14267/2575 and PW395/14268 respectively, while primers LPW12722/12723 amplified the *dcl-2* gene. For screening the clones of pAN7-*dcl-1*, a 1333 bp and a 1386 bp fragments would be amplified from successful transformants using primers LPW14269/2575 and LPW395/14270 respectively, while primers LPW12720/12721 amplified the *dcl-1* gene. For screening the clones of pAN7-*qde-2*, a 1339 bp and a 1414 bp fragments would be amplified from successful transformants using primers LPW17320/2575 and LPW395/17321 respectively, while primers LPW14804/14805 amplified the *qde-2* gene. For screening the clones of *dcl-1* for *dcl^{DKO}*, a 1336 bp and a 1517 bp fragments would be amplified from successful transformants using primers LPW14269/2575 and PW395/14270 respectively, while primers LPW12720/12721 amplified the *dcl-1* gene. Real time qPCR would be used for confirming the *dcl-1*, *dcl-2* and *qde-2* expressions in the corresponding *dcl-1^{KO}*, *dcl-2^{KO}*, *dcl^{DKO}*, *qde-2^{KO}* deletions mutants with the primers on Table 1.

2.8   Animal experiments

2.8.1   Animal strains

Female Balb/C mice of 7-8 weeks old weighing 18-25 g were obtained from the Laboratory Animal Unit, Faculty of Medicine, the University of Hong Kong. Mice were caged under standard conditions regulated day and night length, temperature and humidity. Sterile food and tap water were given to mice *ad libitum*.

2.8.2   Mice challenge

To assess the virulence level of the dcl^{DKO} and qde-2^{KO} mutant strains, mice challenging with the conidia of wild type , dcl^{DKO} and qde-2^{KO} *P. marneffei* strains was performed as followed: Conidia were harvested from *P. marneffei* strains grown on SDA at 25°C for 7-8 days to 1× PBS with 0.05% Tween 20 (Sigma-Aldrich, Missouri, USA). 10 mice per group were challenged with *P. marneffei* conidia by intravenous injection via tail vein at a dosage of 8×10^6 spores per mice using 1ml syringe with 27G needles. Mice mortality was recorded daily for 60 days post-injections and analyzed by Kaplan-Meier method and Log-rank test.

2.9   Intracellular Survival of *P. marneffei* in macrophages

To assess the intracellular survival of qde-2^{KO} mutant strain of *P. marneffei* in macrophages, a human and a murine macrophage cell lines were used. The murine macrophage cell line J774 (Sigma-Aldrich) was maintained in DMEM (Invitrogen) supplemented with 10% fetal bovine serum (FBS) routinely and a human acute monocytic leukemia cell line THP1 (American type culture collection, Manassas,

USA), was maintained in suspension in RPMI 1640 medium (Invitrogen) supplemented with 10% FBS routinely. Cell cultures were kept in an air incubator at 37°C and supplemented with 5% CO_2.

Intracellular survival assays procedures were as followed: J774 macrophages of 4×10^5 cells per well were seeded to 24-well tissue culture plates and 1×10^6 cells per well of THP1 monocytes were seeded to 24-well tissue culture plates. Differentiation of THP1 monocytes into macrophages was induced by the supplementation of 100nM PMA in RPMI 1640 medium. Cell cultures were incubated for 24 h before adding conidia of *P. marneffei*. Fresh culture media were replaced in each well. Conidia at a multiplicity of infection (MOI) of 1 were inoculated to the cell culture in 24-wells plate and incubated in an 37°C, 5% CO2 air incubator for 2 h to allow adhesion and invasion to occur. The macrophages were then washed with 240 U/ml of nystatin (Sigma-Aldrich) in medium to kill the extracellular non-phagocyted conidia. Nystatin was removed and rinsed with warm Hank's Buffered Salt Solution (HBSS) to the macrophages. Fresh warm culture media were added to the macrophages and incubated for 24 h. 1% Triton X-100 (Sigma-Aldrich) were used to lyse cells after 24 h post infection. Cell lysates were serial diluted in 1X PBS and plated on Sabouraud dextrose agar (SDA) for colony forming unit (CFU) count. The CFUs recovered from cell lysates after phagocytosis (2 h post infection) were defined as the initial inocula and set as the baseline for intracellular survival analysis. CFUs recovered at 24 h post infection were taken to calculate the recovery rate of fungal cells. The mean of intracellular survival of conidia was calculated by three independent experiments.

2.10   Hydrogen peroxide killing assay

To assess the protective effect of the $dcl-1^{KO}$, $dcl-2^{KO}$, dcl^{DKO} and $qde-2$ mutant strains against hydrogen peroxide in *P. marneffei*. The conidia of wild type and mutant strains were adjusted to 4×10^3 conidia/ml in 1x PBS with 25 mM hydrogen peroxide (Romero-Martinez, et al., 2000). Aliquots were taken at 5 min intervals and diluted in PBS to minimize hydrogen peroxide activity: 0 min, 5 min, 10 min, 15 min and 20 min. The diluted conidia were plated onto Sabouraud dextrose agar plates at room temperature for CFUs counts.

2.11   Purification of small RNA

To extract small RNA for performing Northern Blotting analysis, *P. marneffei* cultures were grown at mycelial and yeast phases. Small RNA was isolated using small RNA isolation procedures in mirVana miRNA Isolation Kit (Ambion, Austin, TX) combined with Plant Isolation Aid (Ambion, Austin, TX) to remove polysaccharides. About 250mg of mycelia or yeast cells of *P. marneffei* were harvested from BHI broth culture. To each microcentrifuge tube, 600µl Lysis/Binding Buffer and 150µl Plant Isolation Aid were added. The samples were then disrupted with acid-washed glass beads (Sigma, USA) using TissueLyser II (Qiagen, Hilden, Germany) at top speed for two minutes twice with 30 seconds resting interval. Disrupted samples were centrifuged for ten minutes at 4°C. The clear supernatant was transferred to a fresh 1.5 ml tube. One-tenth volume of miRNA Homogenate Additive was added to the supernatant and was left on mix for 10 min. After that, 1:1 volume of Acid-Phenol:Chloroform was added to the lysate before the addition of the miRNA Homogenate Additive. The samples were vortexed using TissueLyser II (Qiagen, Hilden, Germany) at top speed for one minute, followed by centrifugation of 5 min at maximum speed at room temperature. The upper aqueous phase was collected. One-third volume of 100% ethanol was added to the upper aqueous phase and mixed thoroughly. Each mixture was then passed through the Filter Cartridge with 15 sec, 10,000 rpm centrifugation. The filtrate was collected and mixed with two-third volume of 100% ethanol. It was then passed through the Filter Cartridge and the flow-through was discarded. The filter was washed with 700μl miRNA Wash Solution 1 once, then twice with 500μl Wash Solution 2/3 with centrifugation speed of 10,000rpm for 15 sec. The Filter was spun for another 1 min to remove residual fluid and was then allowed to air-dry for at least 2 min. To each dry filter with new Collection Tube, 100μl pre-heated (95°C) nuclease-free water was applied. The elution was then done with spinning for 30 sec at maximum speed. The small RNA was recovered and stored at -80°C.

2.12   Iluminia Solexa Sequencing

2.12.1   Small RNA purification, library preparation and sequencing

To extract small RNA for the library preparation for Illuminia Solexa sequencing, *P. marneffei* cultures were grown at mycelial and yeast phases. Small RNA was isolated following the total RNA isolation procedures of mirVana miRNA Isolation Kit combined with Plant Isoaltion Aid (Ambion, Austin, TX), and digested with DNase (Ambion, Austin, TX) to remove residual DNA contamination that would otherwise interfere with transcriptome analysis. Ribosomal RNAs were removed using RiboMinus Eukaryote Kit for RNA-Seq (Invitrogen, Carlsbad, CA). The rRNA-depleted RNA was concentrated by ethanol precipitation in the presence of glycogen carrier (Amibion, Austin, TX). RNA concentration was determined using a NanoDrop ND-1000 sptrectrophortometer (NanoDrop Technologies, Wilmington, DE, USA). A strand-specific library construction protocol was used to generate template for Illumina DNA sequencing (Hafner, Landgraf et al. 2008). An adenylated 3'-adaptor (5'-rAppAGATCGGAAGAGCGGTTCAGCAGGAATGCCGAG/3ddC/-3') (Integrated DNA Technologies, Coralville, IA) was first ligated to the 3' end of a small RNA fraction (<60nt) by incubating with T4 RNA Ligase 2, truncated (NEB, Ipswich, MA) at 22℃ for 3 h. A biotin-modified adaptor-remover oligonucleotide (5'-2-Bio/rArUrCrGrUrArGrGrCrArCrCrUrGrArArA-3') (Integrated DNA Technologies, Coralville, IA) was added to the ligation mixture to remove excessive 3' adaptors, and incubated at 22℃ for 2.5 h. Both ligated and unligated biotin-modified adaptor-remover oligonucleotides were removed using Dynabeads MyOne Streptavidin C1 (Invitrogen, Carlsbad, CA). The remaining 3' adaptor-ligated small RNAs were precipitated with Pellet Paint (Novagen Inc., Madison, WI), and ligated with 5' adaptor (5'-rArCrArCrUrCrUrUrUrCrCrCrUrArCrArCrGrArCrGrCrUrCrUrUrCrCrGrArUrCrU-3') (Integrated DNA Technologies, Coralville, IA) by incubating with T4 RNA Ligase 1 (NEB, Ipswich, MA) at 22℃ for 3 h. Adaptor-ligated small RNA was reverse transcribed to first-strand cDNA using RT primer (5'- CTCGGCATTCCTGCTGAACCGCTC-3') (Integrated DNA Technologies, Coralville, IA) and SuperScript Double Stranded cDNA Synthesis Kit (Invitrogen, Carlsbad, CA). The cDNA was enriched with 12 PCR cycles using AccuPrime Pfx DNA Polymerase (Invitrogen, Carlsbad, CA) and PCR primers (5'-AATGATACGGCGACCACCGAGATCTACACTCTTTCCCTACACGACGCTCTT

CCGATCT-3' and

5'-CAAGCAGAAGACGGCATACGAGATCGGTCTCGGCATTCCTGCTGAACCGCT
CTTCCGATCT-3') (Integrated DNA Technologies, Coralville, IA). The PCR product
was run on Novex 8% TBE polyacrylamide gel (Invitrogen, Carlsbad, CA) and stained
with SYBR Gold (Invitrogen, Carlsbad, CA). The gel slice containing the 140–190 bp
fragments was excised, and small RNA library was purified by MinElute Gel Extraction
Kit (Qiagen, Valencia, CA). Concentration of gel-purified library was measured by
ND-1000 UV/Vis spectrophotometer (NanoDrop Technologies, Wilmington, DE). Small
RNA library was sequenced on Illumina Genome Analyzer IIx using Illumina
methodology.

2.13   Small RNA analyses

Sequence reads were processed to remove low quality reads, adaptor-dimer
sequences, and nuclear and mitochrondrial rRNA sequences to yield 16,479,305 and
12,754,677 filtered reads for mycelia and yeast phases respectively.

Relative expression levels of milRNA candidates were estimated by normalizing
read counts for each non-redundant small RNA species against RPM (number of reads
per million mapped reads) as mapped to the draft *P. marneffei* PM1 genome sequences
(Woo, Lau et al. 2011). Small RNA sequences between 17-30 nt were selected to identify
perfect matches to the genome using Bowtie (0.12.8) (Langmead, Trapnell et al. 2009).

2.14   Prediction of milRNA candidates

To identify miRNAs candidates, other non-coding RNAs including rRNAs and tRNAs were first excluded. Potential miRNA candidates were predicted with miRDeep (Friedlander, Chen et al. 2008) based on draft *P. marneffei* PM1 genome. The software of miRDeep was chosen because it was the only highthroughput sequencing data miRNA prediction package which allow using custom genomes at that moment. Analysis was performed with the following adjustments: (1) Filtering ubiquitous alignments, keeping only reads that were perfectly mapped to no more than 5 different regions in the genome; (2) Potential precursor sequences were excised from the genome with the size of 250 nt flanking to the sequencing reads; (3) Hybridization temperatures of 25°C and 37°C were used in the script regarding RNAfold for deep sequencing data from mycelial and yeast form of *P. marneffei* respectively. Potential milRNAs were identified with the following criteria: small RNAs that formed a stem-loop structure (hairpin) with flanking sequences (up to 250 nt), as examined by RNAfold in miRDeep package.

2.15   Northern Blot Analyses

Northern blot analysis for the milRNA candidates was performed according to published protocols with modifications (Lau, Woo et al. 2012). Briefly, 10-20 μg of small RNAs was separated on 12% denatured polyacrylamide gel and transferred onto a positively charged nylon membrane (Amersham Biosciences, United Kingdom) with NorthernMax One- Hours Transfer buffer (Ambion) by means of capillary force for 1 h. Crosslinking of RNA to Hybond-NX was performed using a CL-1000 UV Cross-linker (UVP) according to the manufacturer's instructions, followed by baking at 80°C for 2 h..

Hybridization was performed in ULTRAhyb-Oligo hybridization buffer (Ambion) for 3'

digoxigenin (DIG) labeled RNA probes (Sigma-Aldrich, Missouri, USA). The probe

sequences for *PM-milR-M1* is 5' -GUCGAUCAUAAGGCGUUUCUC-DIG-3' and

PM-milR-M2 is 5'-GACUGGCUUUACUAUAGGAC-DIG-3'.

The detection of the DIG-labeled probe on the blot was performed by using DIG

Luminescent Detection kit following the manufacturer's instructions (Roche, Germany).

2.16   Real time qPCR assay

To investigate the expression level of *dcl-1*, *dcl-2* and *qde-2*, real time quantitative

PCR assay was performed as followed : Actin gene of *P. marneffei* strain *PM1* was used

for normalization with primers LPW20631 5'-GAACGTGAAATCGTCCGT -3' and

LPW20160 5'-CACACCTTCTACAACGAGCTCC -3'. The assay was performed using

7900HT Real-Time PCR Thermo Cycler (Applied Biosystems). The reaction mixtures

were prepared according to the manufacturers protocols of FastStart Universal SYBR

Green Master kit (Roche Applied Science, Germany). Briefly, cDNA were amplified for

standard conditions of 45 cycles of 95°C for 15 s, followed by 60°C for 1 min

dissociation step according to the SDS 2.4 software of the Thermo cycler (Applied

Biosystems) was also performed to exclude the possibility of primer-dimer in data

collection steps that may interfere with the results. The qRT-PCT primers for the *dcl-1*,

dcl-2 and *qde-2* are described in Table 1.

2.17   Target Prediction for milRNAs

The potential targets of miRNA candidates were predicted using the predicted gene

71

sequences, including their 5' and 3' UTRs, of the *P. marneffei* strain PM1 and ATCC strain 18442 draft genomes by the RNAhybrid program (Kruger and Rehmsmeier 2006) with or without mismatches or insertions at positions 9-11 of the miRNA and with parameters that encourage complete complementarity at the seed region (positions 2-7 of the miRNA) and (Lewis, Burge et al. 2005).

To classify the predicted targets into functional categories, the predicted protein sequences of the targets were BLASTP against the KOG (Eukaryotic Orthologous Groups of proteins) database with a cutoff identify of 0.5.

CHAPTER 3

FUNCTIONAL CHARACTERIZATION OF DCL-1, DCL-2 AND QDE-2 PROTEINS

3.1   Results

3.1.1   Identification and sequencing analysis of *dcl-1*, *dcl-2* and *qde-2* genes in *P. marneffei*

Using the respective homologues of *N. crassa* for BLAST search of *P. marneffei* strain *PM1* draft genome sequence, two *dcl* genes, *dcl-1* and *dcl-2*, encoding putative Dicer-like proteins and a gene, *qde-2*, encoding a putative Argonaute-like protein were identified (Fig. 8A). Dicer and Argonaute proteins are known to be involved in the biogenesis of miRNAs in animals and plants (Mallory and Vaucheret 2010; Mukherjee, Campos et al. 2013). The *dcl-1* gene is 5,383 bp in length. It has 15 introns of total 889 bp. The resultant mRNA encodes 1,497 amino acid residues with a predicted molecular mass of 170.31 kDa. The *dcl-2* gene is 4,636 bp in length. It has six introns of total 340 bp. The resultant mRNA encodes 1,431 amino acids with a predicted mass of 161.15 kDa. These putative proteins possessed 42% and 32% amino acid identities to the DCL-1 and DCL-2 of *N. crassa* respectively. Both predicted proteins contain all four domains characteristic of the Dicer family. Two RNase III domains are present in the C-terminal region, and a DEAD-box ATP binding domain is present in the N-terminal region (Fig. 8A). In between there are RNA helicase and double stranded RNA binding domains. The

73

qde-2 gene is 3,199 bp in length. It has three introns of total 160 bp. The resultant mRNA encodes 1,012 amino acid residues with a predicted molecular mass of 111.75 kDa. The predicted QDE-2 protein possessed 35% amino acid identity to the QDE-2 of *N. crassa*. It contains two characteristic domains of the argonaute family, PAZ and Piwi domains, and the DUF1785 domain conserved in many argonaute proteins. The domain organization of DCL-1, DCL-2 and QDE-2 of *P. marneffei* is similar to that of the corresponding homologues in *N. crassa* (Catalanotto, Pallotta et al. 2004). The nucleotide sequences of the dcl-1, dcl-2 and qde-2 genes of P. marneffei have been deposited with GenBank under accession no. KC686608, KC686609 and KC686610 respectively.

Our previous study based on mitochondrial genome sequence has shown that *P. marneffei* is phylogenetically more closely related to those of filamentous fungi, including *Aspergillus* species, than yeasts (Woo, Zhen et al. 2003). Phylogenetic analysis of both ITS, another important marker for fungal identification and phylogeny, and *dcl-1* gene showed that the corresponding sequences in *P. marneffei* were most closely related to *Talaromyces stipitatus* (a teleomorph of *Penicillium emmonsii*), *Penicillium chrysogenum* and *Aspergillus* spp. (Fig. 8B). In contrast, phylogenetic analysis of *dcl-2* and *qde-2* genes showed a different evolutionary topology. The *dcl-2* of *P. marneffei* and its homologue in *T. stipitatus* are more closely related to those of the thermal dimorphic pathogenic fungi, *Histoplasma capsulatum*, *Blastomyces dermatitidis*, *Paracoccidioides brasiliensis* and *Coccidioides immitis* than to *P. chrysogenum* and *Aspergillus* spp., suggesting the co-evolution of *dcl-2* among the thermal dimorphic fungi. On the other hand, *qde-2* of *P. marneffei* is most closely related to its homologues in other thermal dimorphic fungi than to that in *T. stipitatus*, *P. chrysogenum* and *Aspergillus* spp..

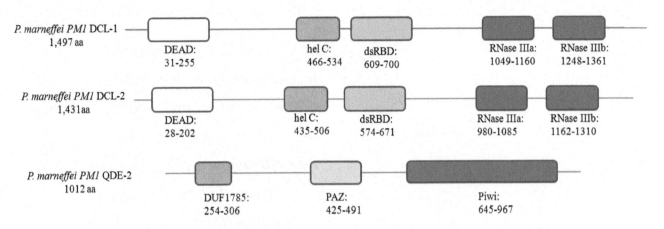

DCL-1

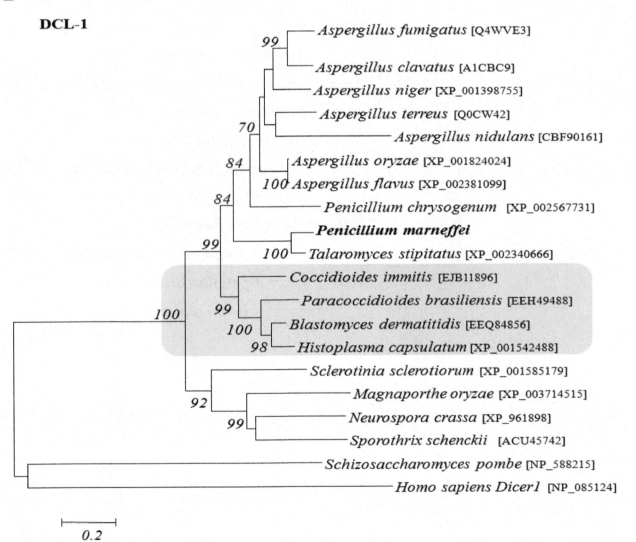

C

DCL-2

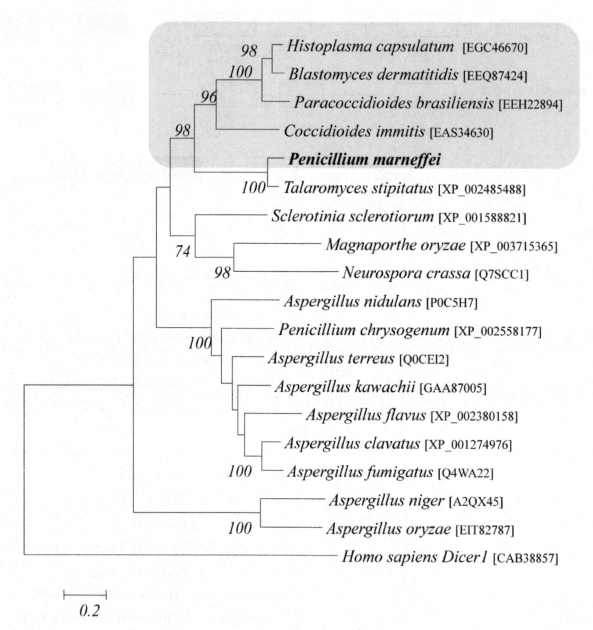

D

QDE-2

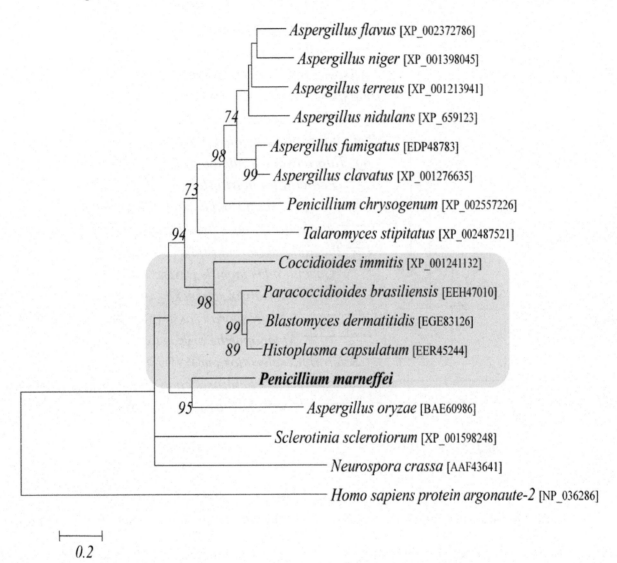

Aspergillus flavus [XP_002372786]

Aspergillus niger [XP_001398045]

Aspergillus terreus [XP_001213941]

Aspergillus nidulans [XP_659123]

Aspergillus fumigatus [EDP48783]

Aspergillus clavatus [XP_001276635]

Penicillium chrysogenum [XP_002557226]

Talaromyces stipitatus [XP_002487521]

Coccidioides immitis [XP_001241132]

Paracoccidioides brasiliensis [EEH47010]

Blastomyces dermatitidis [EGE83126]

Histoplasma capsulatum [EER45244]

Penicillium marneffei

Aspergillus oryzae [BAE60986]

Sclerotinia sclerotiorum [XP_001598248]

Neurospora crassa [AAF43641]

Homo sapiens protein argonaute-2 [NP_036286]

0.2

77

E

ITS

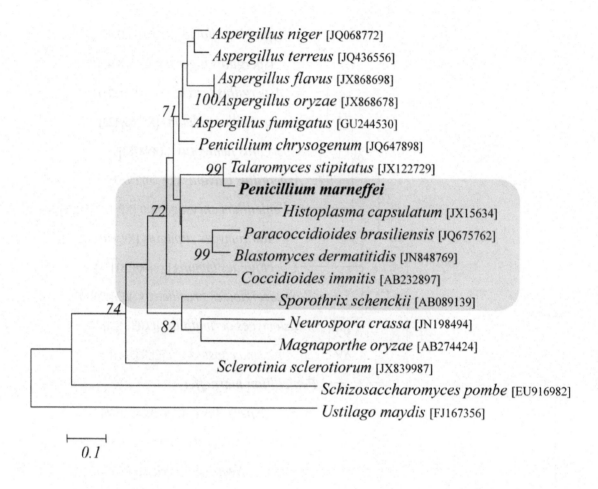

Figure 8. Sequence analysis of *dcl-1, dcl-2* and *qde-2* genes in *P. marneffei*. (A) Predicted domains of Dicer and QDE-2 proteins in *P. marneffei* strain PM1. Black bars represent the full protein sequence. The boxes represent the identified domains, each with its starting and stopping amino acid. Both DCL1 and DCL2 of *P. marneffei* contain a DEAD box, a helicase C domain (hel C), a double stranded RNA binding domain (dsRBD), and two RNase III domains (RNase IIIa and RNase IIIb). QDE-2 contains a PAZ domain ,a Piwi domain and a DUF1785 domains. Phylogenetic tree showing the relationship of

predicted protein sequences of (B) *dcl-1*, (C) *dcl-2*, (D) *qde-2* and ITS of *P. marneffei* to homologues in other fungi constructed by maximum-likelihood method with *Homo sapiens* (DCL-1,DCL-2 and QDE-2) and *Ustilago maydis* (ITS) as the root. The thermal dimorphic pathogenic fungi are highlighted. A total of 914, 764 and 525 amino acid positions for *dcl-1*, *dcl-2* and *qde-2* and 465 nucleotide positions for ITS were included in the analysis respectively. Bootstrap values were calculated as percentages from 1000 replicates and only values ≥70% were shown. The scale bars indicate the estimated number of substitutions per 5, 5, 5 amino acids and 10 bases respectively. Names and accession numbers are given as cited in GenBank database.

3.1.2 Differential mRNA expression of *dcl-1*, *dcl-2* and *qde-2* in mycelial and yeast phases

The mRNA expression level of *dcl-1* in yeast phase was significantly higher than mycelial phase by 25-fold ($P<0.001$ by student t test). In contrast, the mRNA expression levels of *dcl-2* and *qde-2* were higher in mycelial phase than in yeast phase by 7-fold and 2-fold respectively ($P<0.001$ by student t test) (Fig. 9).

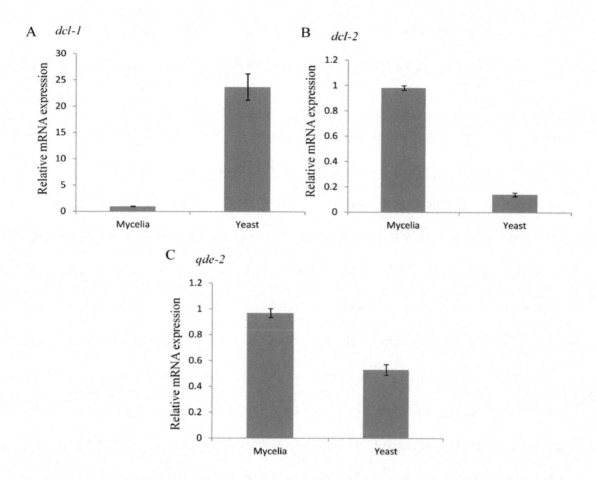

Figure 9. Relative mRNA expression of (A) *dcl-1,* (B) *dcl-2* and (C) *qde-2* genes in mycelial and yeast phase of *P. marneffei* by qRT-PCR. The mRNA expression level of *dcl-1* in yeast phase was significantly higher than mycelial phase by 25-fold ($P<0.001$ by student t test). In contrast, the mRNA expression levels of *dcl-2* and *qde-2* were higher in mycelial phase than in yeast phase by 7-fold and 2-fold respectively ($P<0.001$ by student t test). Results were obtained from five independent experimental replicates ($P<0.001$).

3.1.3   *P. marneffei* knockout mutant strains of *dcl-1*, *dcl-2* and *qde-2*

To study the role of DCL-1, DCL2 and QDE-2, their deletion mutants of *dcl-1^{KO}*, *dcl-2^{KO}*, *dcl^{DKO}*, *qde-2^{KO}* P. *marneffei* strain PM1 were generated. The gene deletion vector – pAN7-*dcl-1*, pAN7-*dcl-2*, pAN7-*qde-2*, pAN8-*dcl-1* were constructed using the plasmid pAN7-1 or pAN8-1 (Fig. 7) as the backbones respectively. The genes *P. marneffei* transformed with linearized pAN7-*dcl-1*, pAN7-*dcl-2*, pAN7-*qde-2* were screened for hygromycin B resistance on SDA supplemented with 150µg/ml hygromycin B. Knockout of *dcl-1*, *dcl-2* and *qde-2* were confirmed by PCR screening using three sets of primers. For screening the clones of pAN7-*dcl-2*, a 1275 bp and a 1547 bp fragments were amplified from successful transformants using primers LPW14267/2575 and PW395/14268 respectively, while primers LPW12722/12723 confirmed the absence of *dcl-2*. For screening the clones of pAN7-*dcl-1*, a 1333 bp and a 1386 bp fragments were amplified from successful transformants using primers LPW14269/2575 and LPW395/14270 respectively, while primers LPW12720/12721 confirmed the absence of *dcl-1*. For screening the clones of pAN7-*qde-2,* a 1339 bp and a 1414 bp fragments were amplified from successful transformants using primers LPW17320/2575 and LPW395/17321 respectively, while primers LPW14804/14805 confirmed the absence of *qde-2*. Double dicers deletion of *dcl^{DKO}* was created by *dcl-2^{KO}* transformed with linearized pAN8-*dcl-1*. It was screened for phyleomycin resistance on SDA supplemented with 100µg/ml phyleomycin. For screening the clones of *dcl-1* for *dcl^{DKO}*, a 1336 bp and a 1517 bp fragments were amplified from successful transformants using primers LPW14269/2575 and PW395/14270 respectively, while primers LPW12720/12721 confirmed the absence of *dcl-1*. Real time qPCR further confirmed undetectable *dcl-1*, *dcl-2* and *qde-2* expressions in the corresponding *dcl-1*^{KO}, *dcl-2*^{KO}, *dcl*^{DKO}, *qde-2*^{KO} deletions mutants.

All deletion mutants exhibited similar growth rates to wild-type strain in both mycelial and yeast phase cultures, although the *dcl*^{DKO} mutant exhibited poor sporulation and reduced red pigment production of smooth colonies compared to wild-type strain upon transition from yeast to mycelial phase on sabouraud agar (Fig. 10).

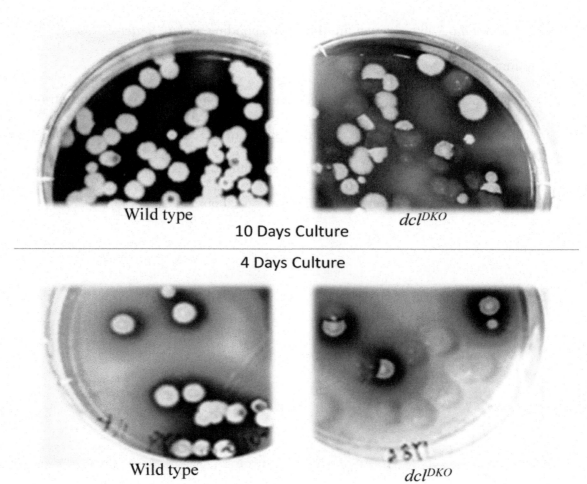

Figure 10. Morphological changes in *dcl^DKO* mutants colonies of *P. marneffei* during yeast to mould transition. The *dcl^DKO* mutant exhibited poor sporulation and reduced red pigment production of smooth colonies compared to wild-type strain upon transition from yeast to mycelial phase on sabouraud agar (Top panel: Older culture of 10 days; Bottom panel: Younger culture of 4 days).

3.1.4 Effect of mice challenged with wild type *P. marneffei* and mutants

To test if the dcl^{DKO} and $qde-2^{KO}$ mutants strain are important in fungal virulence, groups of ten mice were challenged with conidia of *P. marneffei*. The survival of mice after intravenous challenge with wild type *P. marneffei* or the dcl^{DKO} or the $qde-2^{KO}$ mutants on day 60 was summarized in Fig. 11. The survival of mice challenged with the $qde-2^{KO}$ mutant was significantly better than those challenged with wild type *P. marneffei* ($P<0.05$). The survival of mice challenged with the dcl^{DKO} mutant has no difference than those challenged with wild type *P. marneffei*.

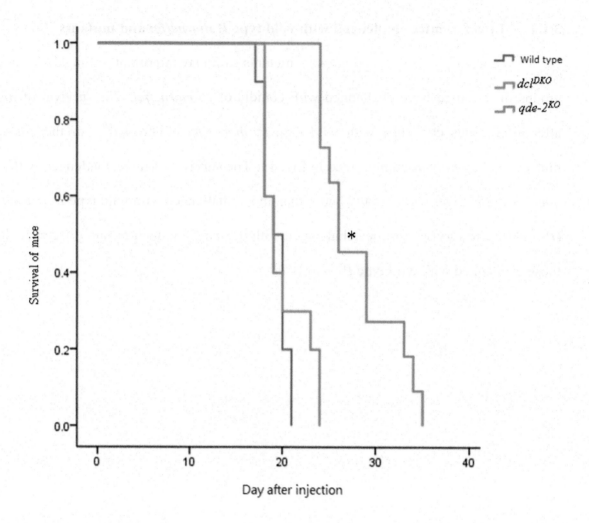

Figure 11. Survival curves of BALB/c mice challenged with wild type, dcl^{DKO} and $qde-2^{KO}$ mutants of *P. marneffei*. The survival of mice challenged with the $qde-2^{KO}$ mutants was significantly better than those challenged with wild type *P. marneffei* ($P<0.05$). The Groups of 10 BALB/c mice were challenged intravenously with 8×10^6 spores. Survival was recorded daily for 60 days.

3.1.5   Survival of *P. marneffei* in macrophages

The results of animal challenging experiment with conidia showed that QDE-2 is related to promote the survival of *P. marneffei* infections in mice, it was hypothesized that such protective function is macrophage related. The main functions of macrophages in innate immunity are to attack and engulf foreign particles, including microbes. It is hypothesized that the QDE-2 may offer survival advantage to *P. marneffei* by protecting the fungus in the host macrophages intracellularly through genes regulation by small RNA. To test the hypothesis, conidia of the wild type and $qde\text{-}2^{KO}$ were recovered from co-cultures of the conidia and J774 or THP1 macrophages after 24 hours post infections. The recovery rate in J774 (n=4) and THP1 (n=3) macrophages of the wild type and mutants 24-hour post-inoculation is summarized in Fig. 12. The recovery rate of the $qde\text{-}2^{KO}$ mutants was lower than the wild type in J774 for 25.7% and THP1 for 17.3% in macrophages respectively ($P<0.05$) (Fig. 12).

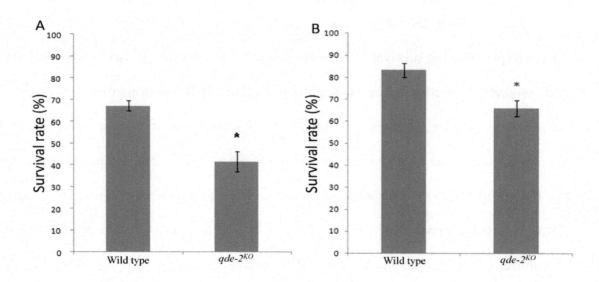

Figure 12. Survival of wild type and *qde-2^{KO}* mutant of *P. marneffei* in J774 and THP1 macrophages. Panels A and B represent the recovery rates of wild type and *qde-2^{KO}* knockout mutant of *P. marneffei* in J774 and THP1 macrophages respectively. Error bars represent as mean ± SEM. Statistical significance between groups is indicated. *: wild type versus *qde-2^{KO}* knockout mutant (*P*<0.05).

3.1.6 Susceptibility to killing by hydrogen peroxide

The relative survival of *P. marneffei* conidia of wild-type and the *qde-2*^{KO} knockout mutant capable of forming visible colonies were calculated and plotted as a function of time of 5, 10, 15 and 20 min incubation in 25 mm hydrogen peroxide. Aliquots were plated on SDA in duplicate to monitor cell viability. Data represent means spore survival ± SEM. (Fig. 13). There are significant lower survival of the *qde-2*^{KO} mutant than wild type mutant in 5 min and 10 min incubation time ($P<0.05$). The sterilizing doses leading to a 50% reduction in survival of the conidia were 9.09 min for wild-type *P. marneffei* and 5.59 min for the *qde-2*^{KO} knockout mutant respectively.

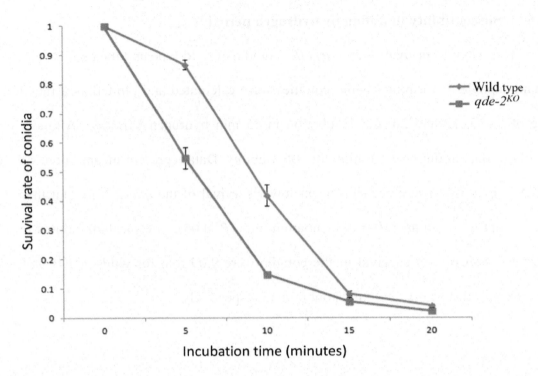

Figure 13. Susceptibility of wild-type *P. marneffei* and its *qde-2*[KO] knockout mutant to hydrogen peroxide. Conidia of wild-type and the *qde-2*[KO] knockout mutant of *P. marneffei* were subjected to killing by hydrogen peroxide for 5, 10, 15 and 20 min. Aliquots were plated on SDA in duplicate to monitor cell viability. There are significant lower survival of the *qde-2*[KO] mutant than wild type mutant in 5 min and 10 min incubation time ($P<0.05$). Data represent means spore survival ± SEM.

3.1.7 Discussion

MicroRNAs and siRNAs are the two important RNAi gene regulators in eukaryotes, including fungi. Gene silencing vectors, such as pSilent-1, have been used as a tool to suppress gene expression in a wide range of fungal species and fungus-like organisms (Nakayashiki and Nguyen 2008). After the transformation of the vectors into the respective fungal species, short hairpin single-stranded RNAs (shRNAs) were transcribed (Nakayashiki, Hanada et al. 2005). The shRNAs were further processed by RNA interference core proteins. In *P. marneffei*, genes such as *alb1* can be knocked down through pSilent-1 transformation (Woo, Tam et al. 2010), implying *P. marneffei* possess all essential RNA interference core proteins to regulate gene expression. In present study, two dicer-like and one argonaute-like QDE-2 proteins were identified in *P. marneffei*. Compared with other ascomycetes, *A. nidulans* has one dicer and one argonaute protein and *Stagonospora nodorum* has four dicers and six argonautes. The numbers of RNAi proteins in fungi are different between species to species. The small RNA machinery may also be different between species to species.

The two *dcl* genes (*dcl-1 and dcl-2*) encoding putative dicer-like proteins and a *qde-2* gene encoding a putative Argonaute-like protein, quelling-deficient-2 (QDE-2), were identified in *P. marneffei* strain PM1 draft genome, which are known to play key roles in the biogenesis of miRNAs and siRNAs (Carthew and Sontheimer 2009). Phylogenetic analysis of both ITS, another important marker for fungal identification and phylogeny, and *dcl-1* gene showed that the corresponding sequences in *P. marneffei* were most closely related to *Talaromyces stipitatus* (a teleomorph of *Penicillium emmonsii*), *Penicillium chrysogenum* and *Aspergillus* spp. (Fig.8). In contrast, phylogenetic analysis

91

of *dcl-2* and *qde-2* genes showed a different evolutionary topology. The *dcl-2* of *P. marneffei* and its homologue in *T. stipitatus* are more closely related to those of the thermal dimorphic pathogenic fungi, *H. capsulatum*, *B. dermatitidis*, *P. brasiliensis* and *C. immitis* than to *P. chrysogenum* and *Aspergillus* spp., suggesting the co-evolution of *dcl-2* among the thermal dimorphic pathogenic fungi. On the other hand, *qde-2* of *P. marneffei* is most closely related to its homologues in other thermal dimorphic fungi than to that in *T. stipitatus*, *P. chrysogenum* and *Aspergillus* spp..

Real-time quantitative PCR results showed that *dcl-1* has higher gene expression in yeast phase than mycelia phase while *dcl-2* and *qde-2* have higher gene expressions in mycelila phase. These suggest *dcl-1* may have important role in yeast phase while *dcl-2* and *qde-2* may have predominantly roles in mycelila phase. Protein levels of *dcl-1*, *dcl-2* and *qde-2* genes could be evaluated to further confirm the observation in mRNA levels. It is because sometimes the mRNA levels could be different from the protein levels. Generating anti-bodies of DCL-1, DCL-2 and QDE-2 are the next step. It is important to study whether *dcl-1*, *dcl-2* or *qde-2* is involved in virulence of *P. marneffei* in order to understand more about the pathogensis of *P. marneffei*.

To test the hypothesis that DCL-2 and QDE-2 are involved in virulence of *P. marneffei*, balb/c mice were challenged with the conidia of *dcl*^{DKO} and *qde-2*^{KO} mutants. Result showed that those mice that were infected with the *dcl*^{DKO} mutant of *P. marneffei* did not show any significant difference when compared with the wild type (Fig. 11), indicating the deletion of the two *dcl* genes did not affect the virulence in *P. marneffei*. This may also imply Dicer regulated milRNAs do not target virulence genes. However, the *qde-2*^{KO} mutant of *P. marneffei* showed a significantly decrease in virulence in mice

92

model. The death of mice that were challenged with qde-2^{KO} conidia were significantly delayed by about 10 days (Fig. 11). This is the first study demonstrated the deletion of an argonaute-like QDE-2 protein (homologue of the slicer Argonaute-2 (Ye, Huang et al. 2011)) in a pathogen resulted in decreased virulence *in vivo*. There are only some suggestions for the connections between Argonaute-2 protein and virulence in other organisms. In protozoan parasite *Entamoeba histolytica*, profiling of Argonaute-2-associated small RNA in both virulent and non-virulent strains suggested some small-RNAs may target virulence-specific genes in virulent strains but not in non-virulent strains (Zhang, Ehrenkaufer et al. 2013). Furthermore, in the human pathogenic bacterium *Streptococcus pneumoniae,* it was demonstrated that many of the identified small non-coding RNAs have important global and niche-specific roles in virulence (Mann, van Opijnen et al. 2012). Also, QDE-2 knockout mutant of *N. crassa* did not show any phenotypic difference with the wild type (Lee, Li et al. 2010). It is hypothesized that if there are QDE-2-associated milRNAs, they may regulate a set of virulence-genes as their targets in *P. marneffei*. It is also hypothesized that the deletion of the *qde-2* gene in *P. marneffei* may diminish the maturation of these virulence-genes targeting milRNAs, resulting in the decrease in virulence in mice model. Identification of QDE-2 regulated milRNAs is important in the future.

The decrease in virulence in mice model of qde-2^{KO} mutant may be due to the higher susceptibility to the oxidative stress inside the macrophages. Phagocytes are the first line of immune defense against *P. marneffei* infection, including monocytes, macrophages, neutrophils, mast cells and dendritic cells. Human and murine macrophage cell lines have been demonstrated to have phagocytic and anti-fungal activities against *P.*

marneffei (Cogliati, Roverselli et al. 1997; Kudeken, Kawakami et al. 1999; Taramelli, Brambilla et al. 2000). In addition, *P. marneffei* can replicate in mononuclear macrophages. However, macrophages are also equipped with antifungal mechanisms to produce reactive nitrogen/oxygen intermediates to combat with the fungal pathogens (Kudeken, Kawakami et al. 2000). Intracellular survival tests were performed to test the survival of *qde-2^KO* conidia in macrophages. The deletion of *qde-2* gene in *P. marneffei* resulted in decreasing survival of *qde-2^KO* conidia in both J774 (Fig. 12A) and THP1 macrophages cell lines (Fig. 12B) and in decreasing resistance to killing by hydrogen peroxide (Fig. 13). While macrophage was suggested to be the most important cell type involved in immunity against *P. marneffei* (Vanittanakom, Cooper et al. 2006), fungi also develop various enzymatic defenses against oxidative stress in host, such as the cytoplasmic superoxide dismutase (SOD), catalases, thiol peroxidases, glutaredoxins, GSH peroxidases, GSH *S*-transferases and methionine sulfoxide reductase (Missall, Lodge et al. 2004). QDE-2 associated milRNAs may target these defensive enzymes against oxidative stress. Therefore, it will be interesting to identify the QDE-2 dependent milRNAs for their role in the pathogenesis of *P. marneffei*.

CHAPTER 4 IDENTIFICATION OF NOVEL MICRORNA-LIKE RNA IN *P. MARNEFFEI*

4.1 Results

4.1.1 Identification of *P. marneffei* small RNAs in by deep sequencing

To examine small RNA species in the two growth phases of *P. marneffei*, cDNA libraries of small RNAs (<60 nt) extracted from mould and yeast cultures respectively were sequenced using an Illumina/Solexa Genome Analyzer IIx. Small RNAs were more abundant in mycelial than yeast phase of *P. marneffei*. The total number of both raw and filtered reads from mycelial and yeast phase was similar (Table 2). However, small RNAs were more abundant in mycelial than yeast phase of *P. marneffei*. We obtained a total of 3,155,063 and 270,782 high-quality, small RNA sequences of size 17-30 nt from mycelial and yeast phases respectively that perfectly match the *P. marneffei* genome. Among these, 362,805 and 56,543 unique small RNA sequences were identified from mycelial and yeast phases respectively (of these, 20,352 of them were in common, identified in both phases) (Fig. 14A). Most of the small RNAs identified from mycelial phase were 17-23 nt long, with the peak at 20-21 nt, and had a strong preference (52.82%) for 5'U (Fig. 14B), a known phenomenon in small RNAs of animals and plants.

4.1.2 Potential milRNAs in *P. marneffei*

Based on the distinguishing features (secondary folding structures and evidences of dicer processing) of known plant and animal miRNAs, 24 potential milRNAs, with flanking sequences forming hairpin secondary structures and at least five reads, were identified (Table 3). Their size distribution was shown in Fig. 14C, with a peak at 21 nt. There was also strong preference for U at their 5' termini (67%, 16 of the 24 milRNA candidates) (Fig. 14D). These include 17 potential milRNAs (2502 reads) in mycelial phase and seven potential milRNAs (232 reads) in yeast phase respectively (Table 3).

Table 2. Analysis of total and small RNA sequences in mycelial and yeast phase of *P. marneffei*

	Total reads	Unique reads
Mycelial		
Raw reads	39,809,400	
Filtered reads	27,914,677	
Adaptors or rRNA reads	11,435,372	
Small RNA reads (17-30nt)	6,910,710	1,077,964
Small RNA reads (17-30nt) mapped to *P. marneffei* genome	3,155,063	362,805
Yeast		
Raw reads	36,999,600	
Filtered reads	28,424,899	
Adaptors or rRNA reads	15,670,222	
Small RNA reads (17-30nt)	768,705	165,545
Small RNA reads (17-30nt) mapped to *P. marneffei* genome	270,782	56,543

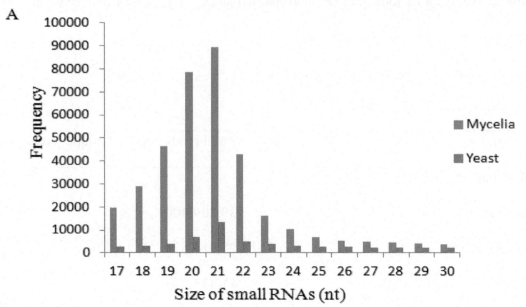

A

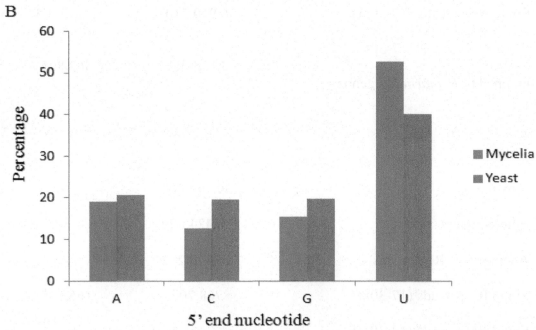

B

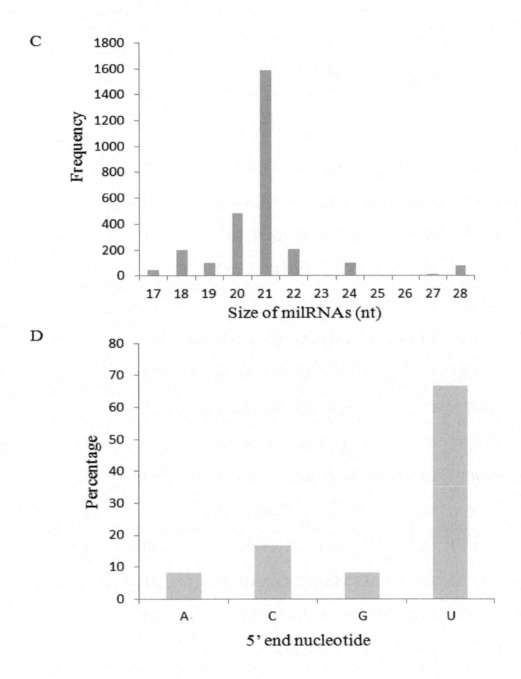

Figure 14. Characterization of small RNAs and milRNAs in *P. marneffei*. (A) Size distribution and (B) Nucleotide frequency of the 5' end of small RNAs in mycelial and yeast phases. (C) Size distribution and (D) Nucleotide frequency of the 5' end of the 24 milRNA candidates.

Table 3. Potential milRNA candidates in mycelial and yeast phase of *P. marneffei*

milRNA	Sequence (5'–3')	Length (nt)	Reads
PM-milR-M1	GAGAAACGCCUUAUGAUCGAC	21	1482
PM-milR-M1*	UGACUCGAAGAGCCUCUA	18	1
PM-milR-M2	GUCCUAUAGUAAAGCCAGUC	20	10
PM-milR-M2*	AUUUCUAGGCUAUAAAAGCUU	21	1
PM-milR-MC3	UGAUAUCAAAGUGGGCUAUC	20	351
PM-milR-MC4	UCAAGUCAACCCUUACUC	18	198
PM-milR-MC5	UUGCUAUGAUGAAAGCUGAGCA	22	127
PM-milR-MC6	AACGUUUAAAUUUCCGAUACAAUU	24	101
PM-milR-MC7	UAGGAUUAGGAUUAGGAUUA	20	97
PM-milR-MC8	UUUCUACAGCUGCUGAACGUC	21	44
PM-milR-MC9	UUGGCGUUGGGUGUAAUUG	19	22
PM-milR-MC10	UCGACUGGCUCACCUGAUGCC	21	14
PM-milR-MC11	UCGAUGUACUUCCUUGUGGA	20	12
PM-milR-MC12	UGUUCAUCGAUCUGCUGUAGA	21	9
PM-milR-MC13	UGCCACUCGAUCAUCUUGGG	20	8
PM-milR-MC14	UAAGAGCUGUACAUAUGUAAG	21	8
PM-milR-MC15	AUCCGGAUCGAGUUAUUCAC	20	8
PM-milR-MC16	CAUAAGGUCGAGAGUCUCGCA	21	6
PM-milR-MC17	UGGCGGACGCGAUGGUGGAGG	21	5
PM-milR-YC1	UGCCAUUGCUAAGUCAAGG	19	76

PM-milR-YC2	CAGCGGUGAUGACAACC	17	47
PM-milR-YC3	CCGCUUCUAAAAUUGCUAGAGC	22	44
PM-milR-YC4	UUGCUAUGAUGAAAGCUGAGCA	22	30
PM-milR-YC5	UUUCUUGUCUACCUUUCGAGU	21	19
PM-milR-YC6	UUCUCGGUGGCGAUGUCCAUU	21	8
PM-milR-YC7	CCUUCAGAUCUGGGCUAUGCCC	22	8

4.1.3   Dicer-dependent biogenesis of milRNA in *P. marneffei*

Northern blot analyses showed the production of milRNAs from two of the predicted milRNA loci, *PM-milR-M1* and *PM-milR-M2*, both from mycelial phase of *P. marneffei*, with their predicted milRNA precursor (pre-milRNA) structures shown in Fig. 15. Seven probes were used, but only two milRNA candidates were visualized. Their predicted precursors were approximately 70-nt and 91-nt in size and had negative folding free energies of -17.86 kcal mol^{-1} and -23.88 kcal mol^{-1} according to RNAfold (http://www.tbi.univie.ac.at/~ivo/RNA/RNAfold.html)   for   *PM-milR-M1*   and *PM-milR-M2* respectively. The majority of small RNA sequences of *PM-milR-M1* and *PM-milR-M2* correspond to one arm of the hairpin (the milRNA arm), with a total of 1482 small RNAs sequenced from *PM-milR-M1* and 10 small RNAs sequenced from *PM-milR-M2* (Table 2). In addition, small RNAs (milRNA*) matched to the complementary arm of the hairpin of *PM-milR-M1* and *PM-milR-M2* were also sequenced, but at much lower frequencies. In contrast to many small RNAs in which the miRNA arm possesses a 5'U position, the milRNA of both *PM-milR-M1* and *PM-milR-M2* have a 5'G position (Fig. 14). The existence of milRNA* and the presence of a 2 nt 3' overhang in these milRNA/milRNA* pairs are strong evidence that they are produced from a Dicer-like enzyme (Fig. 15) (Rajagopalan, Vaucheret et al. 2006). Since loci which produce mature miRNAs and miRNA* sequences are considered miRNA loci, the two loci are tentatively named as *P. marneffei milR-1* (*PM-milR-1*) and *PM-milR-2*. The locus, *PM-milR-1*, was situated within the coding region of a hypothetical protein, whereas *PM-milR-2* was predicted to originate from the opposite strand of a pogo transposable element within a repeat region in the *P. marneffei* genome. The other 22 loci were considered milRNA candidates (named *PM-milR-MC3, MC4...MC17* for milRNA candidates in mycelial phase and *PM-milR-YC1...YC7* for those in yeast phase). These novel milRNAs or milRNA candidates showed no sequence similarity to known miRNAs miRBase Release 19.0 as of January 2013.

To study the expression profile of *PM-milR-M1* and *PM-milR-M2* in mycelial and yeast phases, Northern blot analyses of small RNAs were performed, which confirmed that they were expressed in mycelial (Fig. 15A) but not yeast phase (Fig. 16) of wild-type strain PM1. To assess the role of *dcl-1, dcl-2* and *qde-1* in the biogenesis of *PM-milR-M1* and *PM-milR-M2*, *dcl-1^{KO}, dcl-2^{KO}, dcl^{DKO}* and *qde-2^{KO}* mutants were generated using homologous recombination. All deletion mutants exhibited similar growth rates and phenotypic characteristics to wild-type strain in both mycelial and yeast phase cultures, although the *dcl^{DKO}* mutant exhibited poor sporulation and reduced red pigment production compared to wild-type strain upon transition from yeast to mycelial phase on sabouraud agar (Chapter 3).

Northern blot analysis of *PM-milR-M1* in wild-type and deletion mutants showed that a band corresponding to the mature milRNA product with approximate size of 21 nt was present in wild-type strain, *dcl-1^{KO}* and *qde-2^{KO}* mutants, but was lost in *dcl-2^{KO}* and *dcl^{DKO}* mutants (Fig. 15A). Moreover, a band with approximate size of 70 nt, which matches the size of the predicted precursor of milRNA (pre-milRNA) of *PM-milR-M1*, was present *dcl-2^{KO}* and *dcl^{DKO}* mutants but not in wild-type strain, *dcl-1^{KO}* or *qde-2^{KO}* mutants. In addition, a band of approximately 30 nt is also seen in *dcl-2^{KO}* and *dcl^{DKO}* mutants but not in wild-type strain, *dcl-1^{KO}* or *qde-2^{KO}* mutants, which may represent an intermediate product of the precursor. This suggested that DCL-2 protein is required for the biogenesis of mature milRNA from *PM-milR-M1* and that the band at about 70 nt is likely the pre-milRNA. In the *dcl-1^{KO}* and *qde-2^{KO}* mutants, the levels of mature milRNA were similar to that of wild-type, indicating that DCL-1 and QDE-2 are not required for milRNA production from *PM-milR-M1*. As for *PM-milR-M2*, the band corresponding to its mature milRNA product, with approximate size of 20 nt, was also present in wild-type strain, *dcl-1^{KO}* and *qde-2^{KO}* mutants, but was lost in *dcl-2^{KO}* and *dcl^{DKO}* mutants (Fig. 15A). This suggested that DCL-2 protein is also required for the biogenesis of mature milRNA from *PM-milR-M2*. In the *dcl-1^{KO}* and *qde-2^{KO}* mutants, the levels of mature milRNA were similar to that of wild-type, indicating that DCL-1 and QDE-2 are not required for milRNA production from *PM-milR-M2*.

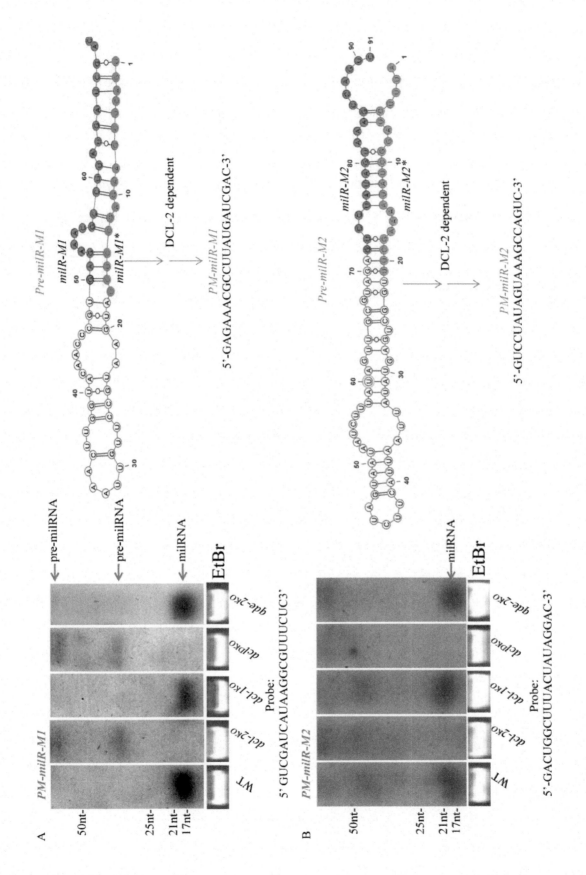

Figure 15. milRNA biogenesis mechanism for *PM-milR-M1* and *PM-milR-2* in *P. marneffei*. (A) Northern blot analyses of small RNA samples in wild-type (WT), *dcl-1^{KO}*, *dcl-2^{KO}*, *dcl^{DKO}* and *qde-2^{KO}* strains of *P. marneffei* showing that the production of milRNA of (A) *PM-milR-M1* and (B) *PM-milR-M2* requires DCL-2 but not DCL-1 or QDE-2. Predicted structures of pre-milRNA of *PM-milR-M1* and *PM-milR-M2*, with their milRNA and paired milRNA* sequences as labeled in red and green respectively, are shown next to the northern blot analyses. The probe sequences used for northern blot analyses are marked.

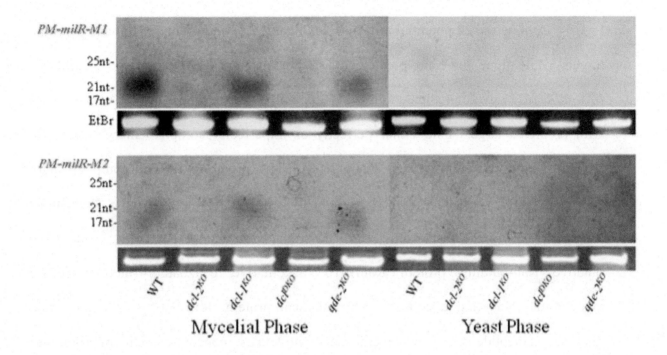

Figure 16. milRNA expressions for *PM-milR-M1* and *PM-milR-M2* in *P. marneffei* mycelial and yeast phases. Northern blot analyses of small RNA samples in wild-type (WT), *dcl-1^{KO}*, *dcl-2^{KO}*, *dcl^{DKO}* and *qde-2^{KO}* strains of *P. marneffei*. *PM-milR-M1* and *PM-milR-M2* were expressed in mycelial but not in yeast phases.

4.1.4   Predicted milRNA targets in *P. marneffei*

Among the 24 potential milRNA candidates, 21 were predicted to have potential targets while three have no predicted targets (Appendix 1). One of the candidates, *PM-milR-MC17*, were predicted to have 353 potential targets. These milRNAs candidates with predicted targets bind either perfectly or imperfectly complementary sequences. However, both *PM-milR-M1* and *PM-milR-M2* were predicted to bind complementary sequences of their targets imperfectly, similar to miRNAs in animals and the filamentous fungus, *N. crassa* (Lee, Li et al. 2010). The predicted targets of *PM-milR-M1* include a putative Ran-binding protein RanBP10, a putative benzoate 4-monooxygenase cytochrome P450 and a conserved hypothetical protein. RanBP10 is a cytoplasmic guanine nucleotide exchange factor that modulates noncentrosomal microtubules involved in mitosis, while cytochrome P450 catalyses diverse reactions in fungal primary and secondary metabolism, and xenobiotic detoxification. As for *PM-milR-M2*, 20 potential targets were predicted, which include 14 transposon or transposable elements and six conserved hypothetical proteins. As shown in Fig. 17, proteins corresponding to the putative targets were classified according to the KOG database. All putative proteins in *P. marneffei* are also classified for comparasion. However, about half of the targets were classified as [S] Function unknown or [R] General function prediction only and no homolog. Most of the remaining targets were classified as the functional category of [Q] Secondary metabolites biosynthesis, transport and catabolism, [J] Translation, ribosomal structure and biogenesis, [O] Posttranslational modification, protein turnover, chaperones, [C] Energy production and conversion, [E] Amino acid transport and metabolism, [D] Cell cycle control, cell division, chromosome partitioning, [A] RNA processing and modification, [T] Signal transduction mechanisms and [U] Intracellular trafficking, secretion, and vesicular transport etc. The KOG distribution of the target proteins was basically similar to all putative proteins in *P. marneffei*, except there were no target proteins being classified as [Y] Nuclear structure and [N] Cell motility.

For all the targets predicted in this study, according to the KOG functional classification, the target genes were classified into three major categories (Fig. 17):

1) Information storage and processing

i. [J] Translation, ribosomal structure and biogenesis, e.g. translation initiation protein Sua5 (target of *PM-milR-MC7*), which is essential for normal translational regulation in yeast (Lin, Ellis et al. 2010).

ii. [A] RNA processing and modification, e.g. DCL-1 (target of *PM-milR-MC7*), dicer-like 1 protein encoded by *dcl-1* gene.

iii. [K] Transcription, e.g. C6 transcription factor (target of *PM-milR-MC6* and *PM-milR-MC10*) which regulates transcription from RNA polymerase II promoter.

iv. [L] Replication, recombination and repair, e.g. topoisomerase family protein TRF4 (target of *PM-milR-MC17*), which has possible role in base excision DNA repair in *S. cerevisiae* (Gellon, Carson et al. 2008).

v. [B] Chromatin structure and dynamics, e.g. transcription factor (Sin3) (target of *PM-milR-MC10*). Deletion of *S. cerevisiae* sin3 resulted in very poor growth on non-fermentable carbon sources and show lower levels of ATP and reduced respiration rates (Barnes, Strunk et al. 2010) .

2) Cellular processes and signaling

i. [D] Cell cycle control, cell division, chromosome partitioning, e.g. nuclear cohesin

109

complex subunit (Psc3) (target of *PM-milR-MC10*), which is involved in meiosis in fission yeast.

ii.   [V] Defense mechanisms, e.g. sugar 1,4-lactone oxidase (target of *PM-milR-YC6*), which is involved in the antioxidant and virulence in *C. albicans* (Huh, Kim et al. 2001).

iii.   [T] Signal transduction mechanisms, e.g. oxysterol binding protein (Orp8) (target of *PM-milR-MC10*), which is suggested to function in lipid metabolism, intracellular lipid transport, membrane trafficking, and cell signaling (Fairn and McMaster 2008).

iv.   [M] Cell wall/membrane/envelop biogenesis, e.g. GPI transamidase component Gpi16 (target of *PM-milR-MC10*), which is a component of the GPI transamidase complex, involved in transfer of GPI to proteins in glycolipid biosynthesis.

v.   [U] Intracellular trafficking, secretion and vesicular transport, e.g. small monomeric GTPase SarA (target of *PM-milr-MC13*), which is involved in intracellular vascular protein transport.

vi.   [O] Posttranslational modification, protein turnover, chaperones, e.g. ubiquitin-protein ligase (Hul4) (target of *PM-milR-MC17*), which is involved in post-transcriptional quality control mechanism limiting inappropriate expression of genetic information in *S. cerevisiae*.

3) Metabolism

i.   [C] Energy production and conversion, e.g. pyruvate dehydrogenase E1 component alpha subunit (target of *PM-milR-YC6*), which is involved in transforming pyruvate into acetyl-CoA in the citric acid cycle to release energy.

ii.   [G] Carbohydrate transport and metabolism, e.g. phosphoglycerate kinase PgkA (target of *PM-milR-MC11*) in glycolysis. There was a study found that the pgkA promoter activity is increased during exponential growth (mostly in mycelium growth) in *P. chrysogenum* (Hoskins and Roberts 1994).

iii. [E] Amino acid transport and metabolism, e.g. acetyltransferase, GNAT family (target of *PM-milR-MC10*). Yeast GCN5 acetylates histones leading to transcription activation, linking histone acetylation and transcriptional regulation directly.

iv. [H] Coenzyme transport and metabolism, e.g. pyridoxine biosynthesis protein (target of *PM-milR-YC7*), which may be involved in growth arrest and cellular response to nutrient limitation in *S. cerevisiae*.

v. [I] Lipid transport and metabolism, e.g. alkaline dihydroceramidase Ydc1 (target of *PM-milR-YC6*), which is involved in ceramide metabolic process. Ceramide is a sphingolipid that play signaling roles in *S. cerevisiae*.

vi. [P] Inorganic ion transport and metabolism, e.g. ammonium transporter (Mep2) (target of *PM-milR-MC17*), which is involved in the ammonium-induced pseudohyphal growth by Mep2-mediated ammonium transport mechanisms in *S. cerevisiae* (Boeckstaens, Andre et al. 2007).

vii. [Q] Secondary metabolites biosynthesis, transport and catabolism, e.g. the fungal secondary metabolite polyketide are synthesized by the polyketide synthases (target of *PM-milR-MC17*). Polyketide has been found to provide survival advantages to *P. marneffei* relate to pigmentation and virulence (Woo, Lam et al. 2012).

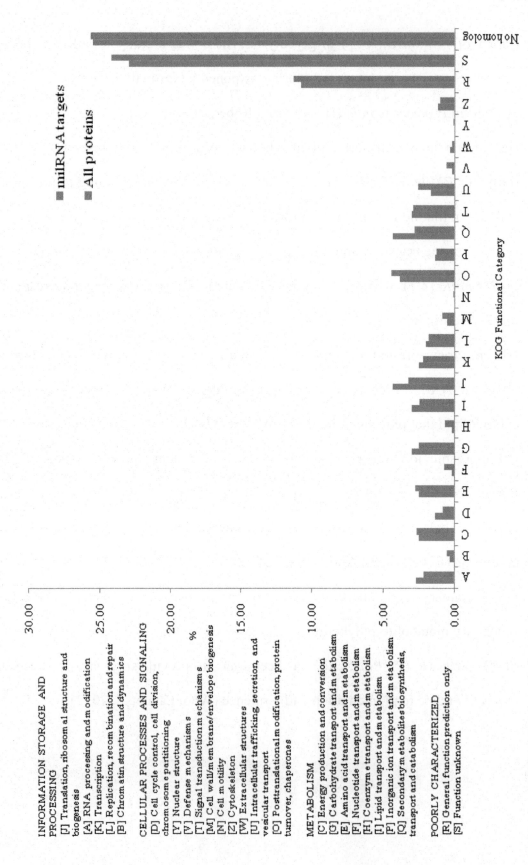

Figure 17. KOG function classification of the predicted target genes.

112

4.1.5 Discussion

This is the first report of the presence of milRNAs in a human dimorphic pathogenic fungus and their differential expression in mycelial and yeast phases. In this study, using high throughput sequencing of small RNAs extracted from mould and yeast cultures of *P. marneffei*, it was shown that small RNAs are more abundantly expressed in mycelial than yeast phase by >10 fold. After exclusion of other non-coding RNAs, a total of 2734 reads were identified as potential milRNA candidates including 17 candidates in mycelial phase and seven in yeast phase, suggesting that milRNAs are differentially expressed in the two growth phases and may be more abundant in mycelial than yeast phase of *P. marneffei*. Two milRNAs, *PM-milR-M1* and *PM-milR-M2*, both expressed in mycelial phase, were confirmed by Northern blot analyses. They share similar characteristics to miRNAs in animals and plants, being dependent on a Dicer-like protein (DCL-2) for production and arisen from highly specific stem-loop RNA precursors. The present results supported that dimorphic fungi may encode milRNAs which are likely conserved regulators of gene expression in diverse eukaryotes including fungi (Bartel 2004).

DCL-2 is likely a conserved protein involved in milRNA biogenesis among thermally dimorphic fungi. Dicer is a member of RNAse III family of nucleases and is responsible for miRNA processing in animals and plants (Bartel 2004). While dicer-like proteins are known to be important for RNAi silencing in various fungi (Kadotani, Nakayashiki et al. 2004; Segers, Zhang et al. 2007; Woo, Tam et al. 2010; Woo, Lam et al. 2012), its role in milRNAs in fungi has been less well studied. A recent study on *N. crassa* has revealed diverse pathways in the generation of milRNAs and

Dicer-independent small interfering RNAs (disiRNAs) (Lee, Li et al. 2010). At least four different mechanisms, that involved a combination of factors, including Dicers and QDE-2, were identified for the production of milRNAs in this filamentous fungus. In this study, the production of *PM-milR-M1* and *PM-milR-M2*, as well as the pre-milRNA of *PM-milR-M2*, was dependent on the presence of DCL-2 but not DCL-1 or QDE-2 in *P. marneffei*. The pre-milRNA of *PM-milR-M2* was not obvious upon Northern blot analyses, which may be due to degradation into small RNAs because of instability. No identifiable homologues of *PM-milR-M1* and *PM–milR-M2* could be identified in animals and plants, which supported the independent evolution of milRNAs in fungi (Lee, Li et al. 2010; Jiang, Yang et al. 2012). On the other hand, homologues of their precursors can be identified in *T. stipitatus* (Appendix 2). Nevertheless, it remains to be determined if such milRNA homologues are also expressed and processed in the same way. The *dcl-2* gene of *P. marneffei* is more closely related to the homologues in other thermal dimorphic fungi than to *P. chrysogenum* and *Aspergillus* spp. in the phylogenetic analysis in Chapter 3.

In contrast to miRNAs from animals and plants which are known to play different functions from multicellular development to stress response, the potential function(s) of milRNAs in fungi remain to be determined. Some miRNAs in plants and animals are known to exhibit temporal or tissue-specific expression patterns (Reinhart, Weinstein et al. 2002; Bartel 2004; Kaufman and Miska 2010). As for fungi, a recent study showed that some milRNAs are differentially expressed in sclerotial development of *S. sclerotiorum* (Zhou, Fu et al. 2012). In *C. neoformans*, milRNAs were shown to cause transgene silencing via the canonical RNAi pathway and proposed to be play a role in regulating transposons and pseudogene expression (Jiang, Yang et al. 2012). In this study, it was shown that the mRNA expression level of *dcl-2* was higher in mycelial than yeast phase, suggesting that DCL-2 may function predominantly in the mycelial phase. This, in turn, may explain why *PM-milR-M1* and *PM–milR-M2* were only expressed in mycelial but not yeast form of *P. marneffei*. Therefore, it is likely that *PM-milR-M1* and *PM-milR-M2* are only produced from DCL-2 and serve important function during mycelial phase. A number of potential targets were predicted for both *PM-milR-M1* and *PM-milR-M2*. For example, the predicted targets of *PM-milR-M1* include RanBP10 and cytochrome P450, while transposon or transposable elements were the predominant predicted targets of *PM-milR-M2*. This suggested that they may regulate cell division, metabolism as well as transposons. On the contrary, the expression level of DCL-1 in yeast phase was 25-fold higher than the mycelial phase, suggesting that DCL-1 may function predominantly in the yeast phase. DCL-1 is another dicer like RNAse III protein that may process precursor milRNA or others small RNAs in yeast phase, but not regulate the *PM-milR-M1* and *PM-milR-M2*. Further studies are required to reveal the exact gene targets, regulatory mechanisms and biological function of milRNAs in *P. marneffei*.

Other than the *PM-milR-M1* and *PM-milR-M2*, 22 potential milRNAs were predicted. Out of the 22 milRNAs, 18 were predicted to target 575 sites, in which 555 were unique target genes. Four milRNAs were predicted to have no targets. Except *PM-milR-MC17* which was predicted to have 353 targets, each milRNA had approximately 13 targets in average. There was evidence that each miRNA has a hundred of target sites in average, suggesting that miRNA may regulate a large number of protein-coding genes (Brennecke, Stark et al. 2005). Other investigations using genome-wide scale computational prediction and biologic data also showed that one miRNA may target tens to hundreds of genes (Krek, Grun et al. 2005; Lim, Lau et al. 2005; Grimson, Farh et al. 2007). It was thus not surprised that the potential milRNAs in *P. marneffei* were predicted to target up to 353 genes.

The predicted targets genes were involved in diverse functional pathway, suggesting the milRNAs may regulate diverse genes in *P. marneffei*. Surprisingly, *dcl-1* was predicted to be the target of *PM-milR-MC17*. The *PM-miilR-MC17* which was expressed in mycelial phase only may suppress *dcl-1* expression in mycelial phase but not in yeast phase, resulting in the higher *dcl-1* expression in yeast than mycelial phase. Besides, *PM-milR-YC6* was predicted to target a DNA helicase RecQ, while RecQ family of DNA helicase is important for maintaining genome integrity. In addition, sugar 1,4-lactone oxidase, the target of *PM-milR-YC6*, is involved in the antioxidant and virulence in *C. albicans* (Huh, Kim et al. 2001). It would be interesting to know if *PM-milR-YC6* is QDE-2 dependent, which may explain why there were reduced virulence and resistance to oxygen intermediates in *P. marneffei* QDE-2^{KO} mutant.

The limitations of this study includes: the lack of a complete genome for the milRNAs and targets predictions, and suitable bioinformatic and experimental tools. Firstly, the draft genome of *P. marneffei* was only in 6x coverage by Sanger sequencing (Woo, Lau et al. 2011), with gaps and unsequenced regions. As a result, there are a number of potential milRNAs that could not be identified in this stage. Future completion of the *P. marneffei* genome should improve the accuracy and sensitivity of the predictions. Secondly, there are no suitable milRNAs prediction pipelines in fungi. milRNA is a recently discovered biomolecule. There are no prediction standards for identifying the potential precursors or targets at this moment. Different prediction methods were used in each milRNAs studies. Standard prediction rules and tools should be suggested after more experimental evidences are available. Functional studies of the milRNAs should be the next step in the milRNA field in fungi. However, there are no suitable protocols for the functional studies of milRNAs while many tools are available in mammalian cells, such as the miRNA inhibitors for silencing specific miRNA or the synthetic miRNA precursors for gain-of-function miRNA experiments. Appropriate experimental protocols must also be developed to facilitate the milRNA research in the future.

CHAPTER 5

CONCLUSIONS AND FUTURE DIRECTIONS

5.1   Conclusions and future directions

P. marneffei is the most important thermal dimorphic fungus causing invasive mycosis in China and Southeast Asia. Despite the findings of diverse genes and mechanisms being involved in dimorphic switching, the key to the genetic circuitry and signally pathways governing the switch is still unknown. Since miRNAs are important gene regulatory molecules in multicellular organisms, it is interesting to define if miRNAs are expressed in different growth phases of *P. marneffei*. Using high-throughput sequencing technology, 24 potential milRNA candidates were identified in *P. marneffei*, which were more abundantly expressed in mycelial than yeast phase. Two genes, *dcl-1* and *dcl-2*, encoding putative Dicer-like proteins and the gene, *qde-2*, encoding Argonaute-like protein, were also identified. Phylogenetic analysis showed that *dcl-2* and *qde-2* of *P. marneffei* was more closely related to the homologues in the other thermal dimorphic pathogenic fungi than to *Penicillium chrysogenum* and *Aspergillus* spp.. *dcl-2* and *qde-2* demonstrated higher mRNA expression levels in mycelial than yeast phase. Northern blot analysis confirmed the expression of two milRNAs, *PM-milR-M1* and *PM-milR-M2*, only in mycelial phase, which was dependent on *dcl-2* but not *dcl-1* or *qde-2*. This study represents the first discovery of milRNAs in thermal dimorphic fungi and demonstrates their differential expression in different growth phases.

Deletion of *qde-2,* but not the two *dcl* genes, was found to decrease the virulence level of *P. marneffei* in mice model. The *qde-2^{KO}* conidia have lower recovery rate both in human and murine macrophages cell line and reduced resistance to hydrogen peroxide than the wild type. QDE-2 was studied widely in *N. crassa*, which can cleave precursor milRNA and associate with milRNAs to regulate gene expression. QDE-2-associated milRNAs may also regulate genes expression, especially virulence genes, in *P. marneffei*. Further investigation of QDE-2-associated milRNAs can provide insights into the correlations between virulence genes and milRNAs. Myc- or His-tagged QDE-2 protein expression cassette can be transformed into the genome of *qde-2^{KO}* mutants of *P. marneffei*. Anti-Myc or Anti-His antibody can be used to purify QDE-2 and its associated small RNAs by immunoprecipitation. The small RNAs can be sequenced and analyzed to reveal the downstream target genes. Then, it will be possible to identify QDE-2-associated small RNAs, which regulate virulence or virulence related genes.

Profiling of small RNAs by deep sequencing of *dcl-1^{KO}, dcl-2^{KO}, dcl^{DKO}, qde-2^{KO}* mutants in both phases in the future can be beneficial for studying the small RNAs maturation pathway in *P. marneffei*, since each knockout mutant can be depleted with a particular set of small RNAs. Studying those sets of small RNAs can provide extra information on the small RNA regulations in *P. marneffei*. It is of interest to know the differences between the small RNA profile of *dcl^{DKO}* or *qde-2^{KO}* and wild type in both yeast and mycelial phases. Deletion of *dcl* or *qde-2* may result in the reduction or overexpression of specific small RNAs in the two phases. In addition, transcriptome analysis of the knockout starins could also be studied. The differentiatlly expressed genes could then be overlapped and assessed with the predicted protein targets. Functional study of the milRNAs can be performed in the future by knocking-out/-down of milRNAs and studying the change of expression levels in their targets. Besides, there is no study investigating the connection between dicers and argonuate proteins in fungi. It is likely that deletions of certain RNAi proteins will lead to a change in the expression level of other RNAi protein to compensate for the loss.

To conclude, the present study extended our knowledge of the milRNAs mechanisms and functions of DCL-2 and QDE-2 in *P. marneffei*. Although our understanding of the functions and the regulatory mechanisms of milRNAs in *P. marneffei* and other thermal dimorphic fungi is far from complete, this study established the foundation for future investigations. The present study revealed the novel DCL-2 dependent biogenesis of milRNAs in *P. marneffei* as well as the differential expression levels of small RNAs in mycelial and yeast phases of the fungus. The relationship between QDE-2 and virulence in *P. marneffei* was also discovered.

APPENDIX 1

Predicted targets of milRNAs in *P. marneffei*

* : perfectly complmentary to targets

milRNAs	target mRNA	site	target
PM-milR-M1	XM_002153120.1| Ran-binding protein (RanBP10), putative, mRNA	1385	2334
PM-milR-M1	XM_002153301.1| conserved hypothetical protein, mRNA	4470	4731
PM-milR-M1	XM_002146036.1| benzoate 4-monooxygenase cytochrome P450, putative, mRNA	267	1200
PM-milR-M2	XM_002144076.1| transposon, putative, mRNA	536	1757
PM-milR-M2	XM_002144493.1| conserved hypothetical protein, mRNA	365	1203
PM-milR-M2	XM_002146057.1| pogo transposable element, putative, mRNA	518	1821
PM-milR-M2	XM_002146378.1| pogo transposable element, putative, mRNA	227	1314
PM-milR-M2	XM_002146381.1| pogo transposable element, putative, mRNA	548	1698
PM-milR-M2	XM_002146475.1| pogo transposable element, putative, mRNA	518	1691
PM-milR-M2	XM_002147154.1| conserved hypothetical protein, mRNA	444	1531
PM-milR-M2	XM_002148112.1| transposon, putative, mRNA	518	1521
PM-milR-M2	XM_002148442.1| conserved hypothetical protein, mRNA	227	1245
PM-milR-M2	XM_002148795.1| transposon, putative, mRNA	518	1668
PM-milR-M2	XM_002149109.1| conserved hypothetical protein, mRNA	227	756
PM-milR-M2	XM_002149110.1| pogo transposable element, putative, mRNA	518	1668
PM-milR-M2	XM_002149111.1| conserved hypothetical protein, mRNA	518	1281
PM-milR-M2	XM_002150101.1| transposon, putative, mRNA	569	1233
PM-milR-M2	XM_002150513.1| pogo transposable element, putative, mRNA	518	1852
PM-milR-M2	XM_002150848.1| transposon, putative, mRNA	518	1302
PM-milR-M2	XM_002150952.1| conserved hypothetical protein, mRNA	478	710
PM-milR-M2	XM_002151776.1| pogo transposable element, putative, mRNA	518	1560
PM-milR-M2	XM_002151777.1| conserved hypothetical protein, mRNA	521	1623
PM-milR-M2	XM_002153191.1| pogo transposable element, putative, mRNA	401	1557
PM-milR-MC3*	XM_002152788.1| conserved hypothetical protein, mRNA	1852	5236
PM-milR-MC3*	XM_002149766.1| conserved hypothetical protein, mRNA	1641	4431
PM-milR-MC3*	XM_002148515.1| conserved hypothetical protein, mRNA	1572	4494
PM-milR-MC3*	XM_002147049.1| conserved hypothetical protein, mRNA	1641	4671
PM-milR-MC3	XM_002147049.1| conserved hypothetical protein, mRNA	1640	4671
PM-milR-MC3	XM_002148515.1| conserved hypothetical protein, mRNA	1571	4494
PM-milR-MC3	XM_002149766.1| conserved hypothetical protein, mRNA	1640	4431
PM-milR-MC3	XM_002151360.1| conserved hypothetical protein, mRNA	1016	1429
PM-milR-MC3	XM_002152788.1| conserved hypothetical protein, mRNA	1851	5236
PM-milR-MC4	no predicted targets		
PM-milR-MC5	XM_002143303.1| hypothetical protein, mRNA	856	956
PM-milR-MC5	XM_002149698.1| protein kinase, putative, mRNA	730	3773
PM-milR-MC6	no predicted targets		
PM-milR-MC7	XM_002144095.1| conserved hypothetical protein, mRNA	1101	1421
PM-milR-MC7	XM_002145998.1| CDP-diacylglycerol-inositol 3-phosphatidyltransferase PIS, mRNA	13	1733
PM-milR-MC7	XM_002146689.1| pyroglutamyl peptidase type I, putative, mRNA	811	1356
PM-milR-MC8	XM_002143560.1| ubiquitin conjugating enzyme, putative, mRNA	3383	3554
PM-milR-MC8	XM_002145926.1| hypothetical protein, mRNA	165	1422
PM-milR-MC8	XM_002147636.1| conserved hypothetical protein, mRNA	1105	4522
PM-milR-MC8	XM_002147898.1| conserved hypothetical protein, mRNA	1302	2949
PM-milR-MC8	XM_002150344.1| tryptophanyl-tRNA synthetase, mRNA	1137	1748
PM-milR-MC8	XM_002150345.1| tryptophanyl-tRNA synthetase, mRNA	1192	1803
PM-milR-MC8	XM_002153352.1| short-chain dehydrogenase/reductase, putative, mRNA	833	1023
PM-milR-MC9	XM_002147966.1| 5-proFAR isomerase His6, putative, mRNA	1208	1596
PM-milR-MC9	XM_002143711.1| DUF221 domain protein, putative, mRNA	1223	3060
PM-milR-MC9	XM_002144412.1| dDENN domain protein, mRNA	477	4125
PM-milR-MC9	XM_002145846.1| acid sphingomyelinase, putative, mRNA	644	1884
PM-milR-MC9*	XM_002147966.1| 5-proFAR isomerase His6, putative, mRNA	1207	1596
PM-milR-MC9	XM_002150722.1| isopropanol dehydrogenase, putative, mRNA	215	1116
PM-milR-MC9	XM_002151377.1| nuclear pore complex protein Nup107, putative, mRNA	14	3207
PM-milR-MC10	XM_002144658.1| GPI transamidase component Gpi16, putative, mRNA	160	1952
PM-milR-MC10	XM_002145491.1| nuclear cohesin complex subunit (Psc3), putative, mRNA	2017	4206
PM-milR-MC10	XM_002145572.1| hypothetical protein, mRNA	1098	1131
PM-milR-MC10	XM_002145754.1| conserved hypothetical protein, mRNA	428	1081
PM-milR-MC10	XM_002146417.1| L-ornithine N5-oxygenase SidA, mRNA	368	2084
PM-milR-MC10	XM_002146889.1| DNA replication initiation factor Cdc45, mRNA	270	3001
PM-milR-MC10	XM_002148504.1| NF-X1 finger transcription factor, putative, mRNA	414	3546
PM-milR-MC10	XM_002148702.1| conserved hypothetical protein, mRNA	996	1418
PM-milR-MC10	XM_002148794.1| urease accessory protein UreG, putative, mRNA	353	1232
PM-milR-MC10	XM_002150625.1| amino acid permease, putative, mRNA	1534	1915
PM-milR-MC10	XM_002152780.1| acetyltransferase, GNAT family, putative, mRNA	324	919

PM-milR-MC10	XM_002152970.1| transcription factor (Sin3), putative, mRNA	3414	4785
PM-milR-MC10	XM_002153528.1| conserved hypothetical protein, mRNA	2775	3763
PM-milR-MC10	XM_002143182.1| conserved hypothetical protein, mRNA	88	1700
PM-milR-MC10	XM_002144551.1| conserved hypothetical protein, mRNA	1203	2472
PM-milR-MC10	XM_002145021.1| phosphotidylinositol kinase Tel1, putative, mRNA	3552	8765
PM-milR-MC10	XM_002145553.1| C6 transcription factor, putative, mRNA	489	2682
PM-milR-MC10	XM_002145900.1| conserved hypothetical protein, mRNA	1730	2289
PM-milR-MC10	XM_002147805.1| UBA/TS-N domain protein, mRNA	766	2833
PM-milR-MC10	XM_002148424.1| aldehyde dehydrogenase, putative, mRNA	238	1410
PM-milR-MC10	XM_002149731.1| fatty acid synthase subunit beta, putative, mRNA	3654	6138
PM-milR-MC10	XM_002150328.1| translation factor pelota, putative, mRNA	1049	1302
PM-milR-MC10	XM_002151211.1| SET domain protein, mRNA	1293	2246
PM-milR-MC10	XM_002152220.1| monocarboxylate permease, putative, mRNA	269	1949
PM-milR-MC10	XM_002152640.1| oxysterol binding protein (Orp8), putative, mRNA	249	2010
PM-milR-MC10	XM_002152641.1| oxysterol binding protein (Orp8), putative, mRNA	249	2406
PM-milR-MC10	XM_002152832.1| conserved hypothetical protein, mRNA	81	1640
PM-milR-MC10	XM_002153112.1| conserved hypothetical protein, mRNA	1037	1602
PM-milR-MC11	XM_002151533.1| phosphoglycerate kinase PgkA, putative, mRNA	1821	2072
PM-milR-MC11	XM_002143366.1| conserved hypothetical protein, mRNA	539	954
PM-milR-MC11	XM_002143532.1| conserved hypothetical protein, mRNA	1685	2076
PM-milR-MC11	XM_002144993.1| ATP dependent RNA helicase (Dbp7), putative, mRNA	290	2440
PM-milR-MC11	XM_002145208.1| conserved hypothetical protein, mRNA	2273	2502
PM-milR-MC11	XM_002145845.1| 6-phosphogluconate dehydrogenase, decarboxylating, mRNA	227	1814
PM-milR-MC11	XM_002148867.1| conserved hypothetical protein, mRNA	109	2589
PM-milR-MC11	XM_002150791.1| nonribosomal peptide synthase, putative, mRNA	21388	23706
PM-milR-MC11*	XM_002151533.1| phosphoglycerate kinase PgkA, putative, mRNA	1820	2072
PM-milR-MC12	XM_002143267.1| conserved hypothetical protein, mRNA	544	1131
PM-milR-MC12	XM_002144529.1| actin cortical patch component, putative, mRNA	756	2062
PM-milR-MC12	XM_002143357.1| MFS sugar transporter, putative, mRNA	1560	1785
PM-milR-MC12	XM_002149005.1| conserved hypothetical protein, mRNA	1220	1281
PM-milR-MC12	XM_002151349.1| alkaline dihydroceramidase Ydc1, putative, mRNA	499	1809
PM-milR-MC12	XM_002152758.1| hypothetical protein, mRNA	467	900
PM-milR-MC12	XM_002153341.1| tubulin-specific chaperone c, putative, mRNA	914	1407
PM-milR-MC13	XM_002143573.1| short-chain dehydrogenase/reductase family protein, putative, mRNA	394	1131
PM-milR-MC13	XM_002146227.1| gamma-tubulin complex component GCP6, putative, mRNA	1911	2994
PM-milR-MC13	XM_002148722.1| F-box and WD repeat-containing protein, mRNA	334	2467
PM-milR-MC13	XM_002150686.1| conserved hypothetical protein, mRNA	431	660
PM-milR-MC13	XM_002144119.1| quinone oxidoreductase, putative, mRNA	837	1120
PM-milR-MC13	XM_002146034.1| conserved hypothetical protein, mRNA	673	1540
PM-milR-MC13	XM_002146249.1| RNA-binding La domain protein, mRNA	914	1389
PM-milR-MC13	XM_002146539.1| conserved hypothetical protein, mRNA	774	1197
PM-milR-MC13	XM_002148831.1| structural maintenance of chromosome complex subunit SmcA, mRNA	759	3566
PM-milR-MC13	XM_002149451.1| short-chain dehydrogenase, putative, mRNA	355	937
PM-milR-MC13	XM_002150156.1| small monomeric GTPase SarA, putative, mRNA	456	1266
PM-milR-MC13	XM_002150157.1| small monomeric GTPase SarA, putative, mRNA	456	1323
PM-milR-MC13	XM_002150325.1| hypothetical protein, mRNA	1883	3123
PM-milR-MC13	XM_002153241.1| cytokinesis protein SepA/Bni1, mRNA	748	5349
PM-milR-MC14	no predicted targets		
PM-milR-MC15	XM_002147735.1| conserved hypothetical protein, mRNA	208	1442
PM-milR-MC15	XM_002150342.1| conserved hypothetical protein, mRNA	1008	3249
PM-milR-MC16	XM_002144804.1| DNA ligase, putative, mRNA	1540	3018
PM-milR-MC16	XM_002147153.1| conserved hypothetical protein, mRNA	686	1596
PM-milR-MC16	XM_002145202.1| fermentation associated protein (Csf1), putative, mRNA	5247	9806
PM-milR-MC16	XM_002149691.1| conserved hypothetical protein, mRNA	260	1392
PM-milR-MC16	XM_002150141.1| 60S ribosomal protein P0, mRNA	245	1160
PM-milR-MC16	XM_002153508.1| conserved hypothetical protein, mRNA	1290	1708
PM-milR-MC17	XM_002143166.1| conserved hypothetical protein, mRNA	547	2290
PM-milR-MC17	XM_002143188.1| UTP-glucose-1-phosphate uridylyltransferase Ugp1, putative, mRNA	613	1982
PM-milR-MC17	XM_002143189.1| UTP-glucose-1-phosphate uridylyltransferase Ugp1, putative, mRNA	719	2088
PM-milR-MC17	XM_002143251.1| gibberellin 20 oxidase, putative, mRNA	73	948
PM-milR-MC17	XM_002143300.1| chitin synthase activator (Chs3), putative, mRNA	24	2925
PM-milR-MC17	XM_002143308.1| beta-glucosidase, putative, mRNA	450	3051
PM-milR-MC17	XM_002143637.1| stress response protein Nst1, putative, mRNA	847	4314
PM-milR-MC17	XM_002143694.1| malate synthase AcuE, mRNA	1495	1880
PM-milR-MC17	XM_002143697.1| 5',5'''-P-1,P-4-tetraphosphate phosphorylase, putative, mRNA	928	1409
PM-milR-MC17	XM_002143913.1| ubiquitin conjugating enzyme (UbcB), putative, mRNA	357	969
PM-milR-MC17	XM_002143926.1| ABC multidrug transporter, putative, mRNA	86	4392
PM-milR-MC17	XM_002144039.1| MFS sugar transporter, putative, mRNA	781	1746
PM-milR-MC17	XM_002144167.1| GPI anchored serine-threonine rich protein, mRNA	528	761
PM-milR-MC17	XM_002144293.1| C2H2 transcription factor Crz1, putative, mRNA	1386	2480
PM-milR-MC17	XM_002144434.1| conserved hypothetical protein, mRNA	7	1633
PM-milR-MC17	XM_002144588.1| conserved hypothetical protein, mRNA	3304	3870
PM-milR-MC17	XM_002144714.1| cysteine-binding protein FliY, putative, mRNA	1387	1878
PM-milR-MC17	XM_002144759.1| RNA helicase/RNAse III, putative, mRNA	2685	4701
PM-milR-MC17	XM_002144806.1| conserved hypothetical protein, mRNA	1125	1755

PM-milR-MC17	XM_002144862.1| hypothetical protein, mRNA	42	888
PM-milR-MC17	XM_002144899.1| mRNA cap methyltransferase, mRNA	688	2103
PM-milR-MC17	XM_002145060.1| conserved hypothetical protein, mRNA	469	1801
PM-milR-MC17	XM_002145201.1| translation elongation factor EF-2 subunit, putative, mRNA	537	2855
PM-milR-MC17	XM_002145286.1| kinesin family protein, mRNA	4760	5689
PM-milR-MC17	XM_002145338.1| MFS transporter, putative, mRNA	1139	2071
PM-milR-MC17	XM_002145353.1| C6 transcription factor, putative, mRNA	1034	2682
PM-milR-MC17	XM_002145384.1| conserved hypothetical protein, mRNA	2389	2828
PM-milR-MC17	XM_002145457.1| Rho guanyl nucleotide exchange factor, putative, mRNA	3854	5908
PM-milR-MC17	XM_002145475.1| tetracycline-efflux transporter, putative, mRNA	1677	1939
PM-milR-MC17	XM_002145478.1| PAP/25A associated domain family, mRNA	1671	3180
PM-milR-MC17	XM_002145525.1| mitochondrial carrier protein (Leu5), putative, mRNA	1230	1945
PM-milR-MC17	XM_002145795.1| conserved hypothetical protein, mRNA	2871	4097
PM-milR-MC17	XM_002145805.1| ribosomal protein S13p/S18e, mRNA	423	783
PM-milR-MC17	XM_002145806.1| ribosomal protein S13p/S18e, mRNA	535	895
PM-milR-MC17	XM_002145831.1| RanGTP-binding protein, mRNA	1191	1998
PM-milR-MC17	XM_002145952.1| cation diffusion facilitator 1, mRNA	850	1496
PM-milR-MC17	XM_002145963.1| poly(A)-binding protein-dependent poly(A) ribonuclease, putative, mRNA	1883	1966
PM-milR-MC17	XM_002145964.1| poly(A)-binding protein-dependent poly(A) ribonuclease, putative, mRNA	130	2676
PM-milR-MC17	XM_002146014.1| conserved hypothetical protein, mRNA	492	1614
PM-milR-MC17	XM_002146259.1| sexual development activator VeA, mRNA	981	2092
PM-milR-MC17	XM_002146301.1| topoisomerase family protein TRF4, putative, mRNA	1834	2336
PM-milR-MC17	XM_002146362.1| DNA excision repair protein Rad16, putative, mRNA	609	3267
PM-milR-MC17	XM_002146577.1| RNA binding protein Jsn1, putative, mRNA	504	3989
PM-milR-MC17	XM_002146594.1| NADH-ubiquinone oxidoreductase 64 kDa subunit, putative, mRNA	254	2085
PM-milR-MC17	XM_002146605.1| short-chain dehydrogenase, putative, mRNA	372	1689
PM-milR-MC17	XM_002146662.1| conserved hypothetical protein, mRNA	175	3148
PM-milR-MC17	XM_002146680.1| RNP domain protein, mRNA	39	1116
PM-milR-MC17	XM_002146725.1| retrograde regulation protein 2, mRNA	954	1749
PM-milR-MC17	XM_002146727.1| thiazole biosynthesis enzyme, mRNA	71	2558
PM-milR-MC17	XM_002146773.1| topisomerase II associated protein (Pat1), putative, mRNA	798	2774
PM-milR-MC17	XM_002146782.1| C6 transcription factor, putative, mRNA	1759	3353
PM-milR-MC17	XM_002146815.1| aldo-keto reductase (AKR13), putative, mRNA	475	1032
PM-milR-MC17	XM_002146960.1| conserved hypothetical protein, mRNA	540	1764
PM-milR-MC17	XM_002146989.1| nonribosomal peptide synthase, putative, mRNA	3631	16992
PM-milR-MC17	XM_002147001.1| mitochondrial cation transporter, putative, mRNA	446	1196
PM-milR-MC17	XM_002147233.1| multidrug resistance protein fnx1, putative, mRNA	292	1765
PM-milR-MC17	XM_002147333.1| transcriptional regulator (Cti6), putative, mRNA	905	2310
PM-milR-MC17	XM_002147343.1| conserved hypothetical protein, mRNA	532	2055
PM-milR-MC17	XM_002147354.1| trehalose-phosphate synthase/phosphatase complex subunit Tps1, putative, mRNA	2115	2240
PM-milR-MC17	XM_002147356.1| AAA family ATPase, putative, mRNA	107	2598
PM-milR-MC17	XM_002147366.1| stress response transcription factor SrrA/Skn7, putative, mRNA	196	1917
PM-milR-MC17	XM_002147383.1| triglyceride lipase-cholesterol esterase, putative, mRNA	478	1828
PM-milR-MC17	XM_002147384.1| triglyceride lipase-cholesterol esterase, putative, mRNA	552	1902
PM-milR-MC17	XM_002147438.1| alpha-1,6-mannosyltransferase subunit (Och1), putative, mRNA	508	1931
PM-milR-MC17	XM_002147472.1| MAP kinase MpkA, mRNA	1638	1976
PM-milR-MC17	XM_002147550.1| cytochrome c oxidase subunit Va, putative, mRNA	119	813
PM-milR-MC17	XM_002147744.1| mitochondrial export translocase Oxa1, putative, mRNA	1574	1906
PM-milR-MC17	XM_002147775.1| signal recognition particle protein SRP54, mRNA	107	1614
PM-milR-MC17	XM_002147794.1| AP-1 adaptor complex subunit mu, putative, mRNA	711	2751
PM-milR-MC17	XM_002147911.1| alcohol dehydrogenase, putative, mRNA	659	1223
PM-milR-MC17	XM_002148132.1| 40S ribosomal protein S3Ae, mRNA	452	1170
PM-milR-MC17	XM_002148177.1| betaine aldehyde dehydrogenase (BadH), putative, mRNA	961	1497
PM-milR-MC17	XM_002148297.1| cytochrome P450 phenylacetate 2-hydroxylase, putative, mRNA	1033	1883
PM-milR-MC17	XM_002148343.1| phosphoglycerate mutase family protein, putative, mRNA	29	525
PM-milR-MC17	XM_002148414.1| glycogen debranching enzyme Gdb1, putative, mRNA	3900	4741
PM-milR-MC17	XM_002148500.1| glucooligosaccharide oxidase, putative, mRNA	1346	1578
PM-milR-MC17	XM_002148546.1| cytosolic phospholipase A2, putative, mRNA	462	2223
PM-milR-MC17	XM_002148648.1| hypothetical protein, mRNA	221	2074
PM-milR-MC17	XM_002148673.1| malate dehydrogenase, NAD-dependent, mRNA	745	1169
PM-milR-MC17	XM_002148740.1| mitochondrial large ribosomal subunit protein L16, putative, mRNA	856	956
PM-milR-MC17	XM_002148752.1| glucan endo-1,3-alpha-glucosidase agn1 precursor, putative, mRNA	167	1850
PM-milR-MC17	XM_002148871.1| conserved hypothetical protein, mRNA	815	1375
PM-milR-MC17	XM_002148882.1| COPII vesicles protein Yip3, putative, mRNA	411	2067
PM-milR-MC17	XM_002149120.1| cytokinesis regulator (Byr4), putative, mRNA	789	3552
PM-milR-MC17	XM_002149188.1| C6 transcription factor, putative, mRNA	1680	2103
PM-milR-MC17	XM_002149215.1| conserved hypothetical protein, mRNA	382	881
PM-milR-MC17	XM_002149253.1| conserved hypothetical protein, mRNA	4343	4600
PM-milR-MC17	XM_002149273.1| conserved hypothetical protein, mRNA	18	1200
PM-milR-MC17	XM_002149363.1| conserved hypothetical protein, mRNA	86	1449
PM-milR-MC17	XM_002149392.1| conserved hypothetical protein, mRNA	805	3626
PM-milR-MC17	XM_002149589.1| conserved hypothetical protein, mRNA	943	1374
PM-milR-MC17	XM_002149771.1| C6 finger domain protein, putative, mRNA	1095	1518
PM-milR-MC17	XM_002149890.1| cell cycle control protein (Cwf22), putative, mRNA	96	2406
PM-milR-MC17	XM_002149958.1| conserved hypothetical protein, mRNA	157	3105

PM-milR-MC17	XM_002150089.1	amino acid transporter, putative, mRNA	1231	1800
PM-milR-MC17	XM_002150212.1	ubiquitin-protein ligase (Hul4), putative, mRNA	564	3735
PM-milR-MC17	XM_002150301.1	UPF0136 domain protein, mRNA	64	389
PM-milR-MC17	XM_002150520.1	60S ribosomal protein L37a, mRNA	464	840
PM-milR-MC17	XM_002150521.1	60S ribosomal protein L37a, mRNA	468	844
PM-milR-MC17	XM_002150522.1	60S ribosomal protein L37a, mRNA	488	864
PM-milR-MC17	XM_002150523.1	60S ribosomal protein L37a, mRNA	648	1024
PM-milR-MC17	XM_002150707.1	conserved hypothetical protein, mRNA	1793	3961
PM-milR-MC17	XM_002150732.1	conserved hypothetical protein, mRNA	828	1539
PM-milR-MC17	XM_002150733.1	GPI anchored protein, putative, mRNA	626	949
PM-milR-MC17	XM_002150734.1	GPI anchored protein, putative, mRNA	629	952
PM-milR-MC17	XM_002150788.1	CCCH zinc finger protein, mRNA	140	2238
PM-milR-MC17	XM_002150807.1	carbamoyl-phosphate synthase, large subunit, mRNA	120	3652
PM-milR-MC17	XM_002150827.1	C6 finger domain protein, putative, mRNA	1458	2832
PM-milR-MC17	XM_002151085.1	serine/threonine-rich protein adg2 precursor, putative, mRNA	499	1413
PM-milR-MC17	XM_002151222.1	proteasome activator subunit 4, putative, mRNA	4823	6537
PM-milR-MC17	XM_002151246.1	glycerol-3-phosphate acyltransferase Sct1, putative, mRNA	1588	2354
PM-milR-MC17	XM_002151266.1	conserved hypothetical protein, mRNA	200	1152
PM-milR-MC17	XM_002151337.1	DNA replication helicase Dna2, putative, mRNA	4355	5013
PM-milR-MC17	XM_002151559.1	DEAD/DEAH box RNA helicase, mRNA	3088	3742
PM-milR-MC17	XM_002151790.1	Rho GTPase activator (Bem3), putative, mRNA	103	4241
PM-milR-MC17	XM_002151839.1	mitochondrial translocase complex component (Tim50), putative, mRNA	208	2142
PM-milR-MC17	XM_002151906.1	SH3 domain protein, mRNA	2646	4172
PM-milR-MC17	XM_002151907.1	SH3 domain protein, mRNA	2636	4162
PM-milR-MC17	XM_002151918.1	cytosolic regulator Pianissimo, putative, mRNA	1842	4068
PM-milR-MC17	XM_002152013.1	alpha-1,3-glucan synthase Ags2, mRNA	3072	7239
PM-milR-MC17	XM_002152063.1	MFS monosaccharide transporter, putative, mRNA	1626	1892
PM-milR-MC17	XM_002152090.1	amino acid transporter, putative, mRNA	1203	2019
PM-milR-MC17	XM_002152200.1	conserved hypothetical protein, mRNA	11258	30287
PM-milR-MC17	XM_002152232.1	conserved hypothetical protein, mRNA	192	1005
PM-milR-MC17	XM_002152310.1	alcohol dehydrogenase, putative, mRNA	188	1359
PM-milR-MC17	XM_002152359.1	acetolactate synthase, putative, mRNA	183	1812
PM-milR-MC17	XM_002152383.1	mitochondrial carrier protein (Rim2), putative, mRNA	392	1282
PM-milR-MC17	XM_002152420.1	conserved hypothetical protein, mRNA	876	1221
PM-milR-MC17	XM_002152478.1	conserved hypothetical protein, mRNA	96	778
PM-milR-MC17	XM_002152558.1	20S cyclosome subunit (APC1/BimE), putative, mRNA	1612	6216
PM-milR-MC17	XM_002152575.1	MAP kinase kinase Ste7, mRNA	1167	2109
PM-milR-MC17	XM_002152704.1	MFS transporter, putative, mRNA	818	1556
PM-milR-MC17	XM_002152730.1	high affinity methionine permease, mRNA	38	1865
PM-milR-MC17	XM_002153168.1	polysaccharide synthase Cps1, putative, mRNA	967	2996
PM-milR-MC17	XM_002153267.1	ABC drug exporter AtrF, mRNA	2936	4605
PM-milR-MC17	XM_002153332.1	threonine synthase Thr4, putative, mRNA	900	1880
PM-milR-MC17	XM_002153455.1	pyruvate dehydrogenase complex component Pdx1, putative, mRNA	36	1261
PM-milR-MC17	XM_002153693.1	hypothetical protein, mRNA	226	1332
PM-milR-MC17	XM_002143098.1	aspergillopepsin A precursor, putative, mRNA	152	1128
PM-milR-MC17	XM_002143164.1	beta-1,4-mannosyltransferase (Alg1), putative, mRNA	458	1392
PM-milR-MC17	XM_002143187.1	membrane bound C2 domain protein (vp115), putative, mRNA	636	4725
PM-milR-MC17	XM_002143192.1	MFS peptide transporter Ptr2, putative, mRNA	1731	2067
PM-milR-MC17	XM_002143202.1	UPF0183 domain protein, mRNA	778	1736
PM-milR-MC17	XM_002143225.1	farnesyl-diphosphate farnesyltransferase, putative, mRNA	143	1798
PM-milR-MC17	XM_002143281.1	glutamate carboxypeptidase Tre2, putative, mRNA	553	3220
PM-milR-MC17	XM_002143297.1	acetamidase, putative, mRNA	1457	1863
PM-milR-MC17	XM_002143309.1	nucleus export ATPase (Elf1), putative, mRNA	3292	3700
PM-milR-MC17	XM_002143339.1	F-box domain protein, mRNA	2269	2640
PM-milR-MC17	XM_002143358.1	COPII vesicle coat protein Sec16, putative, mRNA	3838	5406
PM-milR-MC17	XM_002143377.1	conserved hypothetical protein, mRNA	5742	6236
PM-milR-MC17	XM_002143431.1	ribonuclease P complex subunit Pop1, putative, mRNA	109	2768
PM-milR-MC17	XM_002143530.1	methyltransferase, putative, mRNA	28	918
PM-milR-MC17	XM_002143771.1	conserved hypothetical protein, mRNA	372	2321
PM-milR-MC17	XM_002143822.1	conserved hypothetical protein, mRNA	309	2415
PM-milR-MC17	XM_002143869.1	RTA1 domain protein, putative, mRNA	979	1387
PM-milR-MC17	XM_002143936.1	CP2 transcription factor, putative, mRNA	1070	2886
PM-milR-MC17	XM_002143974.1	ferric-chelate reductase, putative, mRNA	340	2029
PM-milR-MC17	XM_002144007.1	translation elongation factor EF-1 alpha subunit , putative, mRNA	421	1523
PM-milR-MC17	XM_002144018.1	BAG domain protein, mRNA	981	1985
PM-milR-MC17	XM_002144070.1	tRNA-specific adenosine deaminase, putative, mRNA	1557	3645
PM-milR-MC17	XM_002144110.1	conserved hypothetical protein, mRNA	106	1716
PM-milR-MC17	XM_002144340.1	pentatricopeptide repeat protein, mRNA	55	2313
PM-milR-MC17	XM_002144368.1	conserved hypothetical protein, mRNA	479	1081
PM-milR-MC17	XM_002144369.1	conserved hypothetical protein, mRNA	548	1150
PM-milR-MC17	XM_002144442.1	HLH DNA binding domain protein, putative, mRNA	130	1421
PM-milR-MC17	XM_002144448.1	dipeptidyl peptidase, putative, mRNA	2952	3992
PM-milR-MC17	XM_002144449.1	dipeptidyl peptidase, putative, mRNA	2952	3935
PM-milR-MC17	XM_002144450.1	dipeptidyl peptidase, putative, mRNA	2952	3932
PM-milR-MC17	XM_002144520.1	protein disulfide isomerase Pdi1, putative, mRNA	1495	2381

PM-milR-MC17	XM_002144648.1| ATP dependent RNA helicase, putative, mRNA	1518	2358
PM-milR-MC17	XM_002144699.1| cytochrome b5, putative, mRNA	306	437
PM-milR-MC17	XM_002144702.1| conserved hypothetical protein, mRNA	1319	3720
PM-milR-MC17	XM_002144790.1| conserved hypothetical protein, mRNA	740	1703
PM-milR-MC17	XM_002144820.1| AMP dependent CoA ligase, putative, mRNA	738	1887
PM-milR-MC17	XM_002144829.1| polyketide synthase, putative, mRNA	748	5427
PM-milR-MC17	XM_002144875.1| conserved hypothetical protein, mRNA	610	1644
PM-milR-MC17	XM_002144937.1| alcohol dehydrogenase, putative, mRNA	389	1434
PM-milR-MC17	XM_002145111.1| conserved hypothetical protein, mRNA	300	1116
PM-milR-MC17	XM_002145411.1| Ctr copper transporter family protein, mRNA	610	1120
PM-milR-MC17	XM_002145412.1| Ctr copper transporter family protein, mRNA	840	1273
PM-milR-MC17	XM_002145413.1| Ctr copper transporter family protein, mRNA	610	1043
PM-milR-MC17	XM_002145460.1| GTPase activating protein (Gyp2), putative, mRNA	110	3603
PM-milR-MC17	XM_002145569.1| conserved hypothetical protein, mRNA	246	2601
PM-milR-MC17	XM_002145570.1| conserved hypothetical protein, mRNA	246	2660
PM-milR-MC17	XM_002145648.1| NRPS-like enzyme, putative, mRNA	873	3946
PM-milR-MC17	XM_002145786.1| conserved hypothetical protein, mRNA	770	1750
PM-milR-MC17	XM_002145792.1| glutathione-S-transferase theta, GST, putative, mRNA	37	657
PM-milR-MC17	XM_002145796.1| conserved hypothetical protein, mRNA	95	1716
PM-milR-MC17	XM_002145799.1| GTPase activating protein (Evi5), putative, mRNA	1124	2960
PM-milR-MC17	XM_002145830.1| BSD domain protein, mRNA	535	1197
PM-milR-MC17	XM_002145865.1| beta-mannosidase, mRNA	2426	2862
PM-milR-MC17	XM_002145891.1| proline-specific permease, putative, mRNA	1314	1650
PM-milR-MC17	XM_002146007.1| conserved hypothetical protein, mRNA	61	1215
PM-milR-MC17	XM_002146054.1| BTB/POZ domain protein, mRNA	313	1507
PM-milR-MC17	XM_002146065.1| hypothetical protein, mRNA	16	174
PM-milR-MC17	XM_002146079.1| polyketide synthase, putative, mRNA	896	7095
PM-milR-MC17	XM_002146303.1| protein kinase C substrate, putative, mRNA	351	1985
PM-milR-MC17	XM_002146307.1| conserved hypothetical protein, mRNA	521	1337
PM-milR-MC17	XM_002146345.1| conserved hypothetical protein, mRNA	336	3751
PM-milR-MC17	XM_002146346.1| C2H2 zinc finger protein, mRNA	303	3103
PM-milR-MC17	XM_002146367.1| phosphatidylinositol 4-kinase (STT4), putative, mRNA	266	7873
PM-milR-MC17	XM_002146399.1| conserved hypothetical protein, mRNA	735	1581
PM-milR-MC17	XM_002146433.1| C6 transcription factor, putative, mRNA	161	2103
PM-milR-MC17	XM_002146461.1| involucrin repeat protein, mRNA	17201	18527
PM-milR-MC17	XM_002146469.1| O-methylsterigmatocystin oxidoreductase, putative, mRNA	1441	1917
PM-milR-MC17	XM_002146752.1| ribonucleotide reductase small subunit RnrA, putative, mRNA	209	1621
PM-milR-MC17	XM_002146935.1| conserved hypothetical protein, mRNA	6	1658
PM-milR-MC17	XM_002146956.1| conserved hypothetical protein, mRNA	318	1062
PM-milR-MC17	XM_002147089.1| C6 transcription factor, putative, mRNA	189	2248
PM-milR-MC17	XM_002147090.1| C6 transcription factor, putative, mRNA	150	2209
PM-milR-MC17	XM_002147183.1| aminotransferase family protein (LolT), putative, mRNA	1218	1750
PM-milR-MC17	XM_002147259.1| cytosolic large ribosomal subunit protein L7A, mRNA	712	1157
PM-milR-MC17	XM_002147335.1| Woronin body protein HexA, putative, mRNA	1505	1919
PM-milR-MC17	XM_002147461.1| cell wall glucanase (Scw4), putative, mRNA	1616	2188
PM-milR-MC17	XM_002147533.1| conserved hypothetical protein, mRNA	1202	2027
PM-milR-MC17	XM_002147541.1| AMID-like mitochondrial oxidoreductase, putative, mRNA	874	1311
PM-milR-MC17	XM_002147560.1| histone acetylase complex subunit Paf400, putative, mRNA	1460	11574
PM-milR-MC17	XM_002147624.1| DUF907 domain protein, mRNA	69	2827
PM-milR-MC17	XM_002147634.1| developmental regulatory protein WetA, mRNA	1173	4366
PM-milR-MC17	XM_002147660.1| LCCL domain protein, mRNA	1060	2250
PM-milR-MC17	XM_002147749.1| transcription initiation factor TFIID complex 60 kDa subunit, mRNA	156	1793
PM-milR-MC17	XM_002147836.1| dolichyl-phosphate beta-glucosyltransferase, putative, mRNA	223	1576
PM-milR-MC17	XM_002147883.1| conserved hypothetical protein, mRNA	1012	1494
PM-milR-MC17	XM_002147887.1| WD repeat protein, mRNA	375	2486
PM-milR-MC17	XM_002147901.1| importin beta-5 subunit, putative, mRNA	151	3232
PM-milR-MC17	XM_002147944.1| conserved hypothetical protein, mRNA	930	1619
PM-milR-MC17	XM_002147961.1| SNF2 family helicase/ATPase (Ino80), putative, mRNA	2844	8085
PM-milR-MC17	XM_002148028.1| aminopeptidase, putative, mRNA	992	2316
PM-milR-MC17	XM_002148057.1| conserved hypothetical protein, mRNA	1222	1941
PM-milR-MC17	XM_002148071.1| cytochrome P450, putative, mRNA	398	1641
PM-milR-MC17	XM_002148085.1| Golgi membrane protein, putative, mRNA	694	987
PM-milR-MC17	XM_002148160.1| calcium channel subunit Mid1, mRNA	183	2072
PM-milR-MC17	XM_002148173.1| hypothetical protein, mRNA	151	753
PM-milR-MC17	XM_002148186.1| conserved hypothetical protein, mRNA	67	2550
PM-milR-MC17	XM_002148196.1| mitochondrial Hsp70 chaperone (Ssc70), putative, mRNA	398	2670
PM-milR-MC17	XM_002148296.1| aquaporin transporter, putative, mRNA	200	1077
PM-milR-MC17	XM_002148459.1| aminoacyl-tRNA hydrolase, putative, mRNA	489	918
PM-milR-MC17	XM_002148460.1| aminoacyl-tRNA hydrolase, putative, mRNA	469	898
PM-milR-MC17	XM_002148461.1| aminoacyl-tRNA hydrolase, putative, mRNA	469	1005
PM-milR-MC17	XM_002148462.1| aminoacyl-tRNA hydrolase, putative, mRNA	575	1004
PM-milR-MC17	XM_002148475.1| GPI transamidase component PIG-U, putative, mRNA	1041	1431
PM-milR-MC17	XM_002148618.1| transcription factor Tos4, putative, mRNA	753	1952
PM-milR-MC17	XM_002148698.1| conserved hypothetical protein, mRNA	1239	1913
PM-milR-MC17	XM_002148892.1| CFEM domain protein, putative, mRNA	674	896

125

PM-milR-MC17	XM_002148896.1| endoplasmic reticulum calcium ATPase, putative, mRNA	190	3456
PM-milR-MC17	XM_002148922.1| snRNP assembly factor, putative, mRNA	1254	1839
PM-milR-MC17	XM_002149002.1| small nucleolar ribonucleoprotein complex subunit, putative, mRNA	2156	3126
PM-milR-MC17	XM_002149072.1| aminopeptidase, putative, mRNA	3894	4106
PM-milR-MC17	XM_002149082.1| conserved hypothetical protein, mRNA	154	2643
PM-milR-MC17	XM_002149083.1| polyketide synthase, putative, mRNA	344	6429
PM-milR-MC17	XM_002149085.1| Pumilio-family RNA binding repeat domain protein, mRNA	46	2957
PM-milR-MC17	XM_002149122.1| NADH-ubiquinone oxidoreductase, subunit G, putative, mRNA	530	2772
PM-milR-MC17	XM_002149207.1| glucan 1,4-alpha-glucosidase, putative, mRNA	1534	1926
PM-milR-MC17	XM_002149212.1| phospholipid-transporting ATPase (DRS2), putative, mRNA	4501	5154
PM-milR-MC17	XM_002149254.1| glutamate synthase Glt1, putative, mRNA	5115	6784
PM-milR-MC17	XM_002149282.1| 6-phosphofructo-2-kinase 1, mRNA	792	2440
PM-milR-MC17	XM_002149310.1| NADH-ubiquinone oxidoreductase 14 kDa subunit, putative, mRNA	271	716
PM-milR-MC17	XM_002149314.1| 37S ribosomal protein Mrp17, mRNA	304	812
PM-milR-MC17	XM_002149327.1| high-affinity nicotinic acid transporter, putative, mRNA	358	1494
PM-milR-MC17	XM_002149497.1| conserved hypothetical protein, mRNA	144	1693
PM-milR-MC17	XM_002149526.1| cell wall glucanase (Scw11), putative, mRNA	604	2511
PM-milR-MC17	XM_002149579.1| polyketide synthase, putative, mRNA	2727	5265
PM-milR-MC17	XM_002149616.1| conserved hypothetical protein, mRNA	1232	1617
PM-milR-MC17	XM_002149624.1| kinesin family protein, mRNA	2585	5327
PM-milR-MC17	XM_002149673.1| MFS transporter, putative, mRNA	281	1443
PM-milR-MC17	XM_002149674.1| MFS transporter, putative, mRNA	281	1506
PM-milR-MC17	XM_002149874.1| conserved hypothetical protein, mRNA	149	1797
PM-milR-MC17	XM_002149953.1| aspartyl-tRNA synthetase, cytoplasmic, mRNA	690	2856
PM-milR-MC17	XM_002149960.1| NTF2 and RRM domain protein, mRNA	1006	1650
PM-milR-MC17	XM_002149999.1| probable O-sialoglycoprotein endopeptidase, mRNA	49	1522
PM-milR-MC17	XM_002150040.1| DENN (AEX-3) domain protein, mRNA	2148	3385
PM-milR-MC17	XM_002150084.1| 1,3-beta-glucanosyltransferase Gel2, mRNA	790	1637
PM-milR-MC17	XM_002150108.1| acetyl xylan esterase (Axe1), putative, mRNA	508	1117
PM-milR-MC17	XM_002150141.1| 60S ribosomal protein P0, mRNA	792	1160
PM-milR-MC17	XM_002150150.1| SAM domain protein, mRNA	198	2538
PM-milR-MC17	XM_002150176.1| general stress response phosphoprotein phosphatase Psr1/2, putative, mRNA	1891	2627
PM-milR-MC17	XM_002150199.1| NADH-cytochrome b5 reductase, putative, mRNA	449	1313
PM-milR-MC17	XM_002150200.1| NADH-cytochrome b5 reductase, putative, mRNA	513	1377
PM-milR-MC17	XM_002150223.1| cyclin (Pcl1), putative, mRNA	690	1758
PM-milR-MC17	XM_002150296.1| DUF726 domain protein, mRNA	169	3359
PM-milR-MC17	XM_002150421.1| C2H2 transcription factor (Seb1), putative, mRNA	340	2630
PM-milR-MC17	XM_002150430.1| 60S ribosomal protein L25, putative, mRNA	464	1023
PM-milR-MC17	XM_002150476.1| beta-lactamase family protein, mRNA	28	1302
PM-milR-MC17	XM_002150517.1| TBC domain protein, putative, mRNA	1731	2609
PM-milR-MC17	XM_002150525.1| Na/K ATPase alpha 1 subunit, putative, mRNA	830	3502
PM-milR-MC17	XM_002150625.1| amino acid permease, putative, mRNA	1233	1915
PM-milR-MC17	XM_002150643.1| GPI-anchored cell wall beta-1,3-endoglucanase EglC, mRNA	761	1738
PM-milR-MC17	XM_002150702.1| conserved hypothetical protein, mRNA	1322	3694
PM-milR-MC17	XM_002150714.1| conserved hypothetical protein, mRNA	864	1604
PM-milR-MC17	XM_002150793.1| C2H2 finger domain protein, putative, mRNA	885	3779
PM-milR-MC17	XM_002150814.1| origin recognition complex subunit 3, putative, mRNA	1577	2127
PM-milR-MC17	XM_002150889.1| conserved hypothetical protein, mRNA	627	837
PM-milR-MC17	XM_002150900.1| conserved hypothetical protein, mRNA	364	1785
PM-milR-MC17	XM_002150971.1| hypothetical protein, mRNA	20	1335
PM-milR-MC17	XM_002151137.1| polyubiquitin UbiD/Ubi4, putative, mRNA	308	1186
PM-milR-MC17	XM_002151138.1| C6 finger domain protein, putative, mRNA	2158	3173
PM-milR-MC17	XM_002151210.1| NADH-ubiquinone oxidoreductase, subunit F, putative, mRNA	65	1645
PM-milR-MC17	XM_002151261.1| MFS monocarboxylate transporter, putative, mRNA	1247	1639
PM-milR-MC17	XM_002151273.1| conserved hypothetical protein, mRNA	2728	2833
PM-milR-MC17	XM_002151282.1| conserved hypothetical protein, mRNA	1041	3212
PM-milR-MC17	XM_002151306.1| tubulin-specific chaperone, putative, mRNA	1553	1880
PM-milR-MC17	XM_002151316.1| anthranilate phosphoribosyltransferase, putative, mRNA	492	1406
PM-milR-MC17	XM_002151322.1| endosomal peripheral membrane protein (Mon2), putative, mRNA	2047	5214
PM-milR-MC17	XM_002151366.1| MFS multidrug transporter, putative, mRNA	1924	2704
PM-milR-MC17	XM_002151385.1| ammonium transporter (Mep2), putative, mRNA	1227	1870
PM-milR-MC17	XM_002151386.1| MAP kinase kinase kinase SskB, putative, mRNA	1892	4344
PM-milR-MC17	XM_002151550.1| C2H2 transcription factor (Egr2), putative, mRNA	205	624
PM-milR-MC17	XM_002151572.1| hypothetical protein, mRNA	273	951
PM-milR-MC17	XM_002151672.1| eukaryotic translation initiation factor 3 subunit EifCk, putative, mRNA	2	1076
PM-milR-MC17	XM_002151718.1| conserved hypothetical protein, mRNA	100	714
PM-milR-MC17	XM_002151733.1| conserved hypothetical protein, mRNA	123	318
PM-milR-MC17	XM_002151737.1| conserved hypothetical protein, mRNA	643	1268
PM-milR-MC17	XM_002151779.1| SET domain protein, mRNA	2016	4099
PM-milR-MC17	XM_002151780.1| conserved hypothetical protein, mRNA	599	1904
PM-milR-MC17	XM_002151811.1| phosphomannomutase (Sec53), putative, mRNA	342	1163
PM-milR-MC17	XM_002151825.1| sulfate transporter, putative, mRNA	113	1361
PM-milR-MC17	XM_002151904.1| 40S ribosomal protein S17, putative, mRNA	1541	1660
PM-milR-MC17	XM_002151945.1| C2H2 transcription factor (Con7), putative, mRNA	173	2435
PM-milR-MC17	XM_002151946.1| C2H2 transcription factor (Con7), putative, mRNA	173	2291

PM-milR-MC17	XM_002151947.1	C2H2 transcription factor (Con7), putative, mRNA	173	2300
PM-milR-MC17	XM_002151948.1	C2H2 transcription factor (Con7), putative, mRNA	173	2348
PM-milR-MC17	XM_002151949.1	C2H2 transcription factor (Con7), putative, mRNA	173	2421
PM-milR-MC17	XM_002152107.1	Mob1 family protein, mRNA	211	1946
PM-milR-MC17	XM_002152116.1	dimethyladenosine transferase, mRNA	512	1329
PM-milR-MC17	XM_002152303.1	glycosyl transferase, putative, mRNA	2319	3253
PM-milR-MC17	XM_002152305.1	hypothetical protein, mRNA	584	2271
PM-milR-MC17	XM_002152350.1	conserved hypothetical protein, mRNA	1541	1752
PM-milR-MC17	XM_002152567.1	conserved hypothetical protein, mRNA	1042	2946
PM-milR-MC17	XM_002152643.1	cell cycle protein kinase, putative, mRNA	370	1984
PM-milR-MC17	XM_002152713.1	alpha,alpha-trehalose glucohydrolase TreA/Ath1, mRNA	1086	3120
PM-milR-MC17	XM_002152720.1	MFS monocarboxylate transporter, putative, mRNA	25	1317
PM-milR-MC17	XM_002152732.1	beta-1,6-glucanase Neg1, putative, mRNA	970	1500
PM-milR-MC17	XM_002152734.1	DUF1212 domain membrane protein, mRNA	2250	2484
PM-milR-MC17	XM_002152745.1	H /K ATPase alpha subunit, putative, mRNA	318	3482
PM-milR-MC17	XM_002152776.1	plasma membrane channel protein (Aqy1), putative, mRNA	2140	2412
PM-milR-MC17	XM_002152965.1	hypothetical protein, mRNA	464	3516
PM-milR-MC17	XM_002152981.1	conserved hypothetical protein, mRNA	769	1191
PM-milR-MC17	XM_002153056.1	ABC transporter, putative, mRNA	24	4865
PM-milR-MC17	XM_002153098.1	molybdopterin synthase small subunit CnxG, mRNA	17	279
PM-milR-MC17	XM_002153100.1	conserved hypothetical protein, mRNA	266	3573
PM-milR-MC17	XM_002153293.1	hydrolase, alpha/beta fold family protein, mRNA	1601	1677
PM-milR-MC17	XM_002153322.1	MFS transporter, putative, mRNA	936	1987
PM-milR-MC17	XM_002153369.1	short-chain dehydrogenases/reductase, putative, mRNA	447	1032
PM-milR-MC17	XM_002153408.1	sucrose transport protein, putative, mRNA	921	1899
PM-milR-MC17	XM_002153438.1	peroxisome biosynthesis protein (PAS8/Peroxin-6), putative, mRNA	1662	4596
PM-milR-MC17	XM_002153521.1	FHA domain protein, mRNA	434	2379
PM-milR-MC17	XM_002153548.1	RNA polymerase II general transcription and DNA repair factor TFIIH component Tfb5,	46	1151
PM-milR-MC17	XM_002153578.1	conserved hypothetical protein, mRNA	835	2577
PM-milR-MC17	XM_002153589.1	MFS transporter of unkown specificity, mRNA	1049	1633
PM-milR-MC17	XM_002153653.1	hypothetical protein, mRNA	28	399
PM-milR-MC17	XM_002153657.1	conserved hypothetical protein, mRNA	682	1575
PM-milR-MC17	XM_002153659.1	hypothetical protein, mRNA	874	2855
PM-milR-MC17	XM_002153678.1	reverse transcriptase, putative, mRNA	520	1888
PM-milR-YC1	XM_002143780.1	conserved hypothetical protein, mRNA	312	999
PM-milR-YC1	XM_002153194.1	RNA methyltransferase, putative, mRNA	514	1300
PM-milR-YC1	XM_002153466.1	alpha-mannosidase, mRNA	425	3276
PM-milR-YC2	XM_002145664.1	conserved hypothetical protein, mRNA	272	2499
PM-milR-YC3	XM_002145038.1	DUF1264 domain protein, mRNA	982	1155
PM-milR-YC3	XM_002152662.1	histone H2B, mRNA	616	1305
PM-milR-YC3	XM_002144322.1	ubiquitin fusion degradation protein UfdB, putative, mRNA	482	3192
PM-milR-YC3*	XM_002145038.1	DUF1264 domain protein, mRNA	981	1155
PM-milR-YC4	XM_002143303.1	hypothetical protein, mRNA	856	956
PM-milR-YC4	XM_002149698.1	protein kinase, putative, mRNA	730	3773
PM-milR-YC5	XM_002143637.1	stress response protein Nst1, putative, mRNA	1791	4314
PM-milR-YC5	XM_002151779.1	SET domain protein, mRNA	2835	4099
PM-milR-YC5	XM_002143393.1	chromosome segregation protein Cse1, putative, mRNA	2761	3411
PM-milR-YC5	XM_002143583.1	peroxisomal dehydratase, putative, mRNA	1377	1779
PM-milR-YC5	XM_002144121.1	DUF1295 domain protein, mRNA	801	1157
PM-milR-YC5	XM_002146418.1	nonribosomal siderophore peptide synthase, putative, mRNA	2029	15318
PM-milR-YC5	XM_002146580.1	ubiquitin hydrolase L3, mRNA	690	852
PM-milR-YC5	XM_002147049.1	conserved hypothetical protein, mRNA	1457	4671
PM-milR-YC5	XM_002148515.1	conserved hypothetical protein, mRNA	1388	4494
PM-milR-YC5	XM_002148861.1	N,N-dimethylglycine oxidase, mRNA	1248	1479
PM-milR-YC5	XM_002148885.1	beta-galactosidase, putative, mRNA	2968	3000
PM-milR-YC5	XM_002149766.1	conserved hypothetical protein, mRNA	1457	4431
PM-milR-YC5	XM_002150658.1	conserved hypothetical protein, mRNA	413	2346
PM-milR-YC5	XM_002151109.1	transcription factor, putative, mRNA	1895	2605
PM-milR-YC5	XM_002152788.1	conserved hypothetical protein, mRNA	1668	5236
PM-milR-YC6	XM_002144523.1	heterogeneous nuclear ribonucleoprotein HRP1, mRNA	1324	1365
PM-milR-YC6	XM_002145827.1	conserved hypothetical protein, mRNA	693	2073
PM-milR-YC6	XM_002146225.1	nitrite reductase NiiA, mRNA	680	3294
PM-milR-YC6	XM_002146859.1	sugar 1,4-lactone oxidase, putative, mRNA	1574	1890
PM-milR-YC6	XM_002146962.1	nonribosomal peptide synthase, putative, mRNA	7019	16626
PM-milR-YC6	XM_002147380.1	cytochrome c oxidase assembly protein (Pet191), putative, mRNA	818	1220
PM-milR-YC6	XM_002147381.1	cytochrome c oxidase assembly protein (Pet191), putative, mRNA	976	1378
PM-milR-YC6	XM_002148879.1	endoplasmic reticulum DnaJ domain protein Erj5, putative, mRNA	1125	1330
PM-milR-YC6	XM_002151161.1	cell cycle regulatory protein, putative, mRNA	1602	2787
PM-milR-YC6	XM_002151222.1	proteasome activator subunit 4, putative, mRNA	3341	6537
PM-milR-YC6	XM_002152059.1	hypothetical protein, mRNA	1289	1344
PM-milR-YC6	XM_002153707.1	RNA interference and gene silencing protein (Qde2), putative, mRNA	455	3892
PM-milR-YC6	XM_002143093.1	hypothetical protein, mRNA	1612	2094
PM-milR-YC6	XM_002143101.1	conserved hypothetical protein, mRNA	1309	1551
PM-milR-YC6	XM_002143799.1	myo-inositol-phosphate synthase, putative, mRNA	1443	2312
PM-milR-YC6	XM_002143906.1	t-complex protein 1, gamma subunit (Cct3), putative, mRNA	1341	1898

PM-milR-YC6	XM_002144564.1	DNA replication licensing factor Mcm4, putative, mRNA	755	3083
PM-milR-YC6	XM_002144644.1	NRPS-like enzyme, putative, mRNA	2741	3126
PM-milR-YC6	XM_002144825.1	transesterase (LovD), putative, mRNA	945	1337
PM-milR-YC6	XM_002145209.1	KH domain protein, mRNA	369	3491
PM-milR-YC6	XM_002145210.1	chitin synthase ChsE, mRNA	4640	5950
PM-milR-YC6	XM_002145297.1	conserved hypothetical protein, mRNA	225	2658
PM-milR-YC6	XM_002145756.1	polyketide synthase, putative, mRNA	1146	6516
PM-milR-YC6	XM_002146024.1	glutathione oxidoreductase Glr1, putative, mRNA	1248	1942
PM-milR-YC6	XM_002146120.1	oligopeptide transporter, OPT family, putative, mRNA	324	2562
PM-milR-YC6	XM_002146124.1	conserved hypothetical protein, mRNA	2221	3000
PM-milR-YC6	XM_002146186.1	geranylgeranyl diphosphate synthase, mRNA	419	2137
PM-milR-YC6	XM_002146263.1	TMEM1 family protein, putative, mRNA	1032	4496
PM-milR-YC6	XM_002146356.1	condensin complex component cnd2, mRNA	333	2772
PM-milR-YC6	XM_002146368.1	cell-cycle checkpoint protein kinase, putative, mRNA	1115	2416
PM-milR-YC6	XM_002146617.1	sister chromatid separation protein (Src1), putative, mRNA	1993	2301
PM-milR-YC6	XM_002147122.1	hypothetical protein, mRNA	1540	2676
PM-milR-YC6	XM_002147125.1	conserved hypothetical protein, mRNA	286	1065
PM-milR-YC6	XM_002147612.1	conserved hypothetical protein, mRNA	1031	1503
PM-milR-YC6	XM_002147752.1	hypothetical protein, mRNA	1272	1404
PM-milR-YC6	XM_002147840.1	aldo-keto reductase, putative, mRNA	565	1158
PM-milR-YC6	XM_002148534.1	reverse transcriptase, putative, mRNA	476	3789
PM-milR-YC6	XM_002148901.1	enolase/allergen Asp F 22, mRNA	62	1482
PM-milR-YC6	XM_002149014.1	lipase 8 precursor, putative, mRNA	1173	1329
PM-milR-YC6	XM_002149058.1	RNA binding protein Nrd1, putative, mRNA	1188	2363
PM-milR-YC6	XM_002149059.1	RNA binding protein Nrd1, putative, mRNA	1188	1861
PM-milR-YC6	XM_002149171.1	pyruvate dehydrogenase E1 component alpha subunit, putative, mRNA	1026	1410
PM-milR-YC6	XM_002149622.1	MFS lactose permease, putative, mRNA	1605	1641
PM-milR-YC6	XM_002149753.1	hypothetical protein, mRNA	702	2052
PM-milR-YC6	XM_002149763.1	conserved hypothetical protein, mRNA	236	1203
PM-milR-YC6	XM_002149779.1	hypothetical protein, mRNA	667	735
PM-milR-YC6	XM_002149914.1	conserved hypothetical protein, mRNA	556	741
PM-milR-YC6	XM_002149965.1	short-chain dehydrogenase, putative, mRNA	181	999
PM-milR-YC6	XM_002150429.1	mRNA splicing protein (Prp39), putative, mRNA	955	1989
PM-milR-YC6	XM_002150542.1	GPR/FUN34 family protein, mRNA	708	1460
PM-milR-YC6	XM_002150699.1	pre-mRNA splicing helicase, putative, mRNA	1228	6753
PM-milR-YC6	XM_002150730.1	alpha-N-acetylglucosaminidase, putative, mRNA	523	2797
PM-milR-YC6	XM_002150808.1	conserved hypothetical protein, mRNA	1387	2004
PM-milR-YC6	XM_002151562.1	conserved hypothetical protein, mRNA	596	747
PM-milR-YC6	XM_002152173.1	hypothetical protein, mRNA	181	939
PM-milR-YC6	XM_002152267.1	zinc-binding oxidoreductase ToxD, putative, mRNA	285	1399
PM-milR-YC6	XM_002152358.1	conserved hypothetical protein, mRNA	830	1545
PM-milR-YC6	XM_002152698.1	bZIP transcription factor HacA, mRNA	392	1629
PM-milR-YC6	XM_002152778.1	conserved hypothetical protein, mRNA	743	1633
PM-milR-YC6	XM_002152806.1	MFS sugar transporter, putative, mRNA	1628	2274
PM-milR-YC6	XM_002152917.1	hypothetical protein, mRNA	1390	2859
PM-milR-YC6	XM_002153137.1	mRNA binding post-transcriptional regulator (Csx1), putative, mRNA	414	1875
PM-milR-YC6	XM_002153254.1	conserved hypothetical protein, mRNA	1575	1644
PM-milR-YC6	XM_002153336.1	Coatomer subunit alpha, putative, mRNA	2002	4070
PM-milR-YC6	XM_002153601.1	protein disulfide isomerase, putative, mRNA	369	1294
PM-milR-YC6	XM_002153619.1	DNA helicase recq, putative, mRNA	982	4695
PM-milR-YC7	XM_002143822.1	conserved hypothetical protein, mRNA	5	2415
PM-milR-YC7	XM_002143824.1	dihydroxy acid dehydratase Ilv3, putative, mRNA	21	1925
PM-milR-YC7	XM_002145052.1	Apc13 domain protein, mRNA	352	588
PM-milR-YC7	XM_002146490.1	conserved hypothetical protein, mRNA	2234	2374
PM-milR-YC7	XM_002146809.1	conserved hypothetical protein, mRNA	236	3447
PM-milR-YC7	XM_002146810.1	conserved hypothetical protein, mRNA	236	3546
PM-milR-YC7	XM_002146914.1	conserved hypothetical protein, mRNA	871	1207
PM-milR-YC7	XM_002147290.1	protein transport protein Sec24, putative, mRNA	65	2816
PM-milR-YC7	XM_002148448.1	phosphoserine aminotransferase, mRNA	1268	1585
PM-milR-YC7	XM_002149613.1	cytochrome P450, putative, mRNA	239	501
PM-milR-YC7	XM_002150352.1	WD repeat protein, mRNA	3421	4044
PM-milR-YC7	XM_002150581.1	EF hand domain protein, mRNA	1781	3043
PM-milR-YC7	XM_002151274.1	GINS complex subunit Psf3, putative, mRNA	793	880
PM-milR-YC7	XM_002151275.1	GINS complex subunit Psf3, putative, mRNA	855	942
PM-milR-YC7	XM_002152109.1	conserved hypothetical protein, mRNA	357	1928
PM-milR-YC7	XM_002143209.1	conserved hypothetical protein, mRNA	243	954
PM-milR-YC7	XM_002144014.1	conserved hypothetical protein, mRNA	872	1389
PM-milR-YC7	XM_002144498.1	ubiquitin hydrolase, putative, mRNA	2432	2555
PM-milR-YC7	XM_002144574.1	translation initiation protein Sua5, mRNA	1024	1506
PM-milR-YC7	XM_002144776.1	DNA repair and transcription protein (Xab2), putative, mRNA	2436	2769
PM-milR-YC7	XM_002145143.1	conserved hypothetical protein, mRNA	2255	9215
PM-milR-YC7	XM_002145188.1	aromatic aminotransferase Aro8, putative, mRNA	1573	1908
PM-milR-YC7	XM_002145227.1	conserved hypothetical protein, mRNA	1016	1092
PM-milR-YC7	XM_002146750.1	WD repeat protein, mRNA	185	2293
PM-milR-YC7	XM_002147163.1	conserved hypothetical protein, mRNA	456	1598

128

PM-milR-YC7	XM_002147859.1	pyridoxine biosynthesis protein, mRNA	173	1179
PM-milR-YC7	XM_002148040.1	alanine racemase family protein, putative, mRNA	815	1015
PM-milR-YC7	XM_002149657.1	alpha-1,6-mannosyltransferase subunit, putative, mRNA	5388	5838
PM-milR-YC7	XM_002150001.1	conserved hypothetical protein, mRNA	895	1507
PM-milR-YC7	XM_002150338.1	conserved hypothetical protein, mRNA	139	1113
PM-milR-YC7	XM_002150449.1	monocarboxylate permease, putative, mRNA	309	1200
PM-milR-YC7	XM_002150790.1	ABC multidrug transporter, putative, mRNA	2402	5003
PM-milR-YC7	XM_002151401.1	calcium channel subunit Cch1, mRNA	543	6791
PM-milR-YC7	XM_002152324.1	conserved hypothetical protein, mRNA	1989	2386
PM-milR-YC7	XM_002152713.1	alpha,alpha-trehalose glucohydrolase TreA/Ath1, mRNA	489	3120
PM-milR-YC7	XM_002152722.1	chlorohydrolase family protein, mRNA	145	1564
PM-milR-YC7	XM_002153429.1	hypothetical protein, mRNA	530	714

APPENDIX 2

milRNA	Precursor Length (nt)	Free Energy kcal mol^{-1}	Precursor sequences 5'->3'	Identities (Coverage) to *T. stipitatus*,
PM-milR-M1	70	-17.86	UGACUCGAAGAGCCUCUAUGAAUGCCUUGUUAAACUUGGUACAACCCGUGAGAAACGCCUUAUG AUCGAC	86% (100%)
PM-milR-M2	91	-23.88	AUUUCUAGGCUAUAAAAGCUUUGGCUGAGUAUAUUAAUUACUUCUAGUAAUAAUCUUUAUAGU UGCGUAGAGUC	87% (100%)
PM-milR-MC3	59	-18.53	UAUACCACUUUAUACCAUCCUAUAAUUCAGAUAUUGGUAUGAUAUCAAAGUGGGCUAUC	No identities
PM-milR-MC4	45	-12.05	CUAAUGGAUUUGAUGUAGCUGCAGUAAUCAAGUCAACCCUUACUC	No identities
PM-milR-MC5	94	-25.71	UUGCUAUGAUGAAAGCUGAGCAUAUGAACCAACGCGCCGGUUGCCUUUGGCCACUGUACUCCGU	No identities
PM-milR-MC6	76	-24.32	ACUCAGAUUACUC GUUGGCGGAGAUCUUACACGUUUUUCCGGACUUUUUAUUUCUAUGUGCUUGUUAACGUUUAAAU	90% (92%)
PM-milR-MC7	101	-33.4	UUCCGAUACAAUU UCACGGGAUUAGGAUUAGGAUUAGGAUUAGGAUUAGGAUUAGGAUUAGGAUUAGGAUUAGGAU	No identities
PM-milR-MC8	75	-41.92	UAGGAUUAGGAUU CGUCCAGCAGCUGUGGAAUACUUCUUCGCGGGCAACCUAUUCCACUCAAGUAGUUUUCUACAGC	No identities
PM-milR-MC9	121	-42.45	UGCUGAACGUC AUUGCCUUUUUAGCUAAUGGUGGGAUUACUUUUGAAUCAUGCAAGUUGGGUCUAGGAUUAAGG AUCGUUAUUCUUAUGACUUUGCAUCCGUUUAUCUUGCUUUUGGCGUUGGGGUGUAAUUG	79% (42%)
PM-milR-MC10	83	-31.43	UCGACUGGCUCACCUGAUGCCUGACUUUACCCUUACGCAUCUUGAAAGGCUACCAAGUGAGGUC	76% (95%)
PM-milR-MC11	55	-22.23	AAAGGAAUUAUGAGCCUUC UUGAGACGAGGAAUCGAGACUCGAAAGAGAUUAAAUCGAUGUACUUCCUUGUGGA	82% (98%)
PM-milR-MC12	105	-49.03	UACGGUUGGAUUGCCUUGCAACUUGUGUCGAUACAGAGCCUAGAUUCCAAGACAUUGGAAGUGG	No identities
PM-milR-MC13	45	-15.27	GUCAUGGUGCCAACAAGUUGUGUUCAUCGAUCUGCUGUAGA CCGACUCGAGCUGUUCGCUGAGCUGUGCCACUCGAUCAUCUUGGG	No identities
PM-milR-MC14	63	-36.41	UACAUAUGUAAGAGCUGUACAUAUGUAAGAGUUCUACAUAUGUAAGAGCUGUACAUAUGUAAG	85% (100%)
PM-milR-MC15	54	-20.16	GAAUAGCUUCGCAGCCACUGGAUUAGUGCCUUUCAUCCGGAUCGAGUUAUUCAC	94% (98%)
PM-milR-MC16	59	-23.93	GGAGACGUGACGCACUUGAGAGAUAUUUUGUGGCAUCUCAUAAGGUCGAGAGUCUCGCA	No identities
PM-milR-MC17	51	-21.05	UGGCGGACGCGAUGGUGGAGGAGCCGACGACGACGCGUUCGGGACGCGUAA	92% (96%)
PM-milR-YC1	80	-25.8	UGCCAUUGCUAAGUCAAGGCUUCUUCCUGUGCAUUUUCUUGCCGCUCAAUGGGAGUUUUGUCUG	95% (100%)
PM-milR-YC2	71	-16.8	UUACAGCUUUGGUAGA UUGUUUUACAUUUGUUUCGAUAGUUCUACAAGCCUGAAAACCAGGCUUCUAUUUCAGCGGUGAU	No identities
PM-milR-YC3	77	-23.7	GACAACC CCGCUUCUAAAAUUGCUAGAGCUUGCCGUUUCCGAAAUACCAUUUCACCAGGACGAGCAAGUGU	99% (100%)
PM-milR-YC4	94	-17.3	GGACAGAGAAGCA UUGCUAUGAUGAAAGCUGAGCAUAUGAACCAACGCGCCGGUUGCCUUUGGCCACUGUACUCCGU	No identities
PM-milR-YC5	55	-21.2	ACUCAGAUUACUCUGUUUUUGUUCAUUGAUU UUUCUUGUCUACCUUUCGAGUUGUUUCUAACAGUUCGAAAGGCAUUCGAGAAAGG	95% (100%)
PM-milR-YC6	78	-28.1	UUCUCGGUGGCGAUGUCCAUUUAGCAGCCCUCGGUCGAUUCUAUUCGAAAGUGAGCUUGAAUAU	85% (94%)
PM-milR-YC7	71	-19.4	CCCCAUCGAGAACG GUAUCGCACACUCUGAGCAAAAUGAGCAUUCAUCAGAUACAGUUCAUUUCCUUCAGAUCUGGGC UAUGCCC	84% (87%)

REFERENCES

Aleman, L. M., J. Doench, et al. (2007). "Comparison of siRNA-induced off-target RNA and protein effects." RNA **13**(3): 385-395.

Allen, E., Z. Xie, et al. (2005). "microRNA-directed phasing during trans-acting siRNA biogenesis in plants." Cell **121**(2): 207-221.

Ambrose, J. A., R. P. Onders, et al. (2001). "Pneumoperitoneum upregulates preproendothelin-1 messenger RNA." Surgical endoscopy **15**(2): 183-188.

Andrianopoulos, A. (2002). "Control of morphogenesis in the human fungal pathogen *Penicillium marneffei*." Int J Med Microbiol **292**(5-6): 331-347.

Arasu, P., B. Wightman, et al. (1991). "Temporal regulation of *lin-14* by the antagonistic action of two other heterochronic genes, *lin-4* and *lin-28*." Genes & development **5**(10): 1825-1833.

Axtell, M. J., J. O. Westholm, et al. (2011). "Vive la difference: biogenesis and evolution of microRNAs in plants and animals." Genome Biol **12**(4): 221.

Bagga, S., J. Bracht, et al. (2005). "Regulation by *let-7* and *lin-4* miRNAs results in target mRNA degradation." Cell **122**(4): 553-563.

Barnes, V. L., B. S. Strunk, et al. (2010). "Loss of the SIN3 transcriptional corepressor results in aberrant mitochondrial function." BMC biochemistry **11**: 26.

Bartel, D. P. (2004). "MicroRNAs: genomics, biogenesis, mechanism, and function." Cell **116**(2): 281-297.

Bartel, D. P. (2009). "MicroRNAs: target recognition and regulatory functions." Cell **136**(2): 215-233.

Baumberger, N. and D. C. Baulcombe (2005). "*Arabidopsis* ARGONAUTE1 is an RNA Slicer that selectively recruits microRNAs and short interfering RNAs." Proceedings of the National Academy of Sciences of the United States of America **102**(33): 11928-11933.

Behm-Ansmant, I., J. Rehwinkel, et al. (2006). "mRNA degradation by miRNAs and GW182 requires both CCR4:NOT deadenylase and DCP1:DCP2 decapping complexes." Genes Dev **20**(14): 1885-1898.

Bhardwaj, S., A. Shukla, et al. (2007). "Putative structure and characteristics of a red water-soluble pigment secreted by *Penicillium marneffei*." Med Mycol **45**(5): 419-427.

Blackwell, M. (2011). "The fungi: 1, 2, 3 ... 5.1 million species?" American journal of botany **98**(3): 426-438.

Boeckstaens, M., B. Andre, et al. (2007). "The yeast ammonium transport protein Mep2 and its positive regulator, the Npr1 kinase, play an important role in normal and pseudohyphal growth on various nitrogen media through retrieval of excreted ammonium." Molecular microbiology **64**(2): 534-546.

Bohnsack, M. T., K. Czaplinski, et al. (2004). "Exportin 5 is a RanGTP-dependent dsRNA-binding protein that mediates nuclear export of pre-miRNAs." RNA **10**(2): 185-191.

Borradori, L., J. C. Schmit, et al. (1994). "Penicilliosis *marneffei* infection in AIDS." J Am Acad Dermatol **31**(5 Pt 2): 843-846.

Boutet, S., F. Vazquez, et al. (2003). "*Arabidopsis* HEN1: a genetic link between endogenous miRNA controlling development and siRNA controlling transgene silencing and virus resistance." <u>Curr Biol</u> **13**(10): 843-848.

Boyce, K. J. and A. Andrianopoulos (2007). "A p21-activated kinase is required for conidial germination in *Penicillium marneffei*." <u>PLoS Pathog</u> **3**(11): e162.

Boyce, K. J. and A. Andrianopoulos (2007). "A p21-activated kinase is required for conidial germination in *Penicillium marneffei*." <u>PLoS pathogens</u> **3**(11): e162.

Boyce, K. J., M. J. Hynes, et al. (2001). "The CDC42 homolog of the dimorphic fungus *Penicillium marneffei* is required for correct cell polarization during growth but not development." <u>Journal of bacteriology</u> **183**(11): 3447-3457.

Boyce, K. J., M. J. Hynes, et al. (2003). "Control of morphogenesis and actin localization by the *Penicillium marneffei* RAC homolog." <u>Journal of cell science</u> **116**(Pt 7): 1249-1260.

Boyce, K. J., M. J. Hynes, et al. (2005). "The Ras and Rho GTPases genetically interact to co-ordinately regulate cell polarity during development in *Penicillium marneffei*." <u>Molecular microbiology</u> **55**(5): 1487-1501.

Boyce, K. J., M. J. Hynes, et al. (2005). "The Ras and Rho GTPases genetically interact to co-ordinately regulate cell polarity during development in *Penicillium marneffei*." <u>Mol Microbiol</u> **55**(5): 1487-1501.

Boyce, K. J., L. Schreider, et al. (2009). "In vivo yeast cell morphogenesis is regulated by a p21-activated kinase in the human pathogen *Penicillium marneffei*." <u>PLoS pathogens</u> **5**(11): e1000678.

Boyce, K. J., L. Schreider, et al. (2009). "In vivo yeast cell morphogenesis is regulated by a p21-activated kinase in the human pathogen *Penicillium marneffei*." <u>PLoS Pathog</u> **5**(11): e1000678.

Boyce, K. J., L. Schreider, et al. (2011). "The two-component histidine kinases DrkA and SlnA are required for in vivo growth in the human pathogen *Penicillium marneffei*." <u>Molecular microbiology</u> **82**(5): 1164-1184.

Brennecke, J., A. Stark, et al. (2005). "Principles of microRNA-target recognition." <u>PLoS biology</u> **3**(3): e85.

Brodersen, P., L. Sakvarelidze-Achard, et al. (2008). "Widespread translational inhibition by plant miRNAs and siRNAs." <u>Science</u> **320**(5880): 1185-1190.

Brodersen, P. and O. Voinnet (2009). "Revisiting the principles of microRNA target recognition and mode of action." <u>Nature reviews. Molecular cell biology</u> **10**(2): 141-148.

Calin, G. A., C. D. Dumitru, et al. (2002). "Frequent deletions and down-regulation of micro- RNA genes *miR15* and *miR16* at 13q14 in chronic lymphocytic leukemia." <u>Proceedings of the National Academy of Sciences of the United States of America</u> **99**(24): 15524-15529.

Canovas, D. and A. Andrianopoulos (2006). "Developmental regulation of the glyoxylate cycle in the human pathogen *Penicillium marneffei*." <u>Mol Microbiol</u> **62**(6): 1725-1738.

Cao, L., C. M. Chan, et al. (1998). "MP1 encodes an abundant and highly antigenic cell wall mannoprotein in the pathogenic fungus *Penicillium marneffei*." <u>Infect Immun</u> **66**(3): 966-973.

Cao, L., D. L. Chen, et al. (1998). "Detection of specific antibodies to an antigenic mannoprotein for diagnosis of *Penicillium marneffei* penicilliosis." <u>J Clin</u>

Microbiol **36**(10): 3028-3031.

Capponi, M., G. Segretain, et al. (1956). "[Penicillosis from *Rhizomys sinensis*]." <u>Bull Soc Pathol Exot Filiales</u> **49**(3): 418-421.

Carthew, R. W. and E. J. Sontheimer (2009). "Origins and Mechanisms of miRNAs and siRNAs." <u>Cell</u> **136**(4): 642-655.

Catalanotto, C., M. Pallotta, et al. (2004). "Redundancy of the two dicer genes in transgene-induced posttranscriptional gene silencing in *Neurospora crassa*." <u>Molecular and cellular biology</u> **24**(6): 2536-2545.

Chaiwarith, R., N. Charoenyos, et al. (2007). "Discontinuation of secondary prophylaxis against penicilliosis *marneffei* in AIDS patients after HAART." <u>AIDS</u> **21**(3): 365-367.

Chan, Y. F. and T. C. Chow (1990). "Ultrastructural observations on *Penicillium marneffei* in natural human infection." <u>Ultrastruct Pathol</u> **14**(5): 439-452.

Chariyalertsak, S., T. Sirisanthana, et al. (1996). "Seasonal variation of disseminated *Penicillium marneffei* infections in northern Thailand: a clue to the reservoir?" <u>J Infect Dis</u> **173**(6): 1490-1493.

Chariyalertsak, S., K. Supparatpinyo, et al. (2002). "A controlled trial of itraconazole as primary prophylaxis for systemic fungal infections in patients with advanced human immunodeficiency virus infection in Thailand." <u>Clin Infect Dis</u> **34**(2): 277-284.

Chariyalertsak, S., P. Vanittanakom, et al. (1996). "*Rhizomys sumatrensis* and *Cannomys badius*, new natural animal hosts of *Penicillium marneffei*." <u>J Med Vet Mycol</u> **34**(2): 105-110.

Chen, K. and N. Rajewsky (2006). "Natural selection on human microRNA binding sites inferred from SNP data." <u>Nature genetics</u> **38**(12): 1452-1456.

Chim, C. S., C. Y. Fong, et al. (1998). "Reactive hemophagocytic syndrome associated with *Penicillium marneffei* infection." <u>Am J Med</u> **104**(2): 196-197.

Chiu, Y. L. and T. M. Rana (2003). "siRNA function in RNAi: a chemical modification analysis." <u>RNA</u> **9**(9): 1034-1048.

Chu, C. Y. and T. M. Rana (2006). "Translation repression in human cells by microRNA-induced gene silencing requires RCK/p54." <u>PLoS biology</u> **4**(7): e210.

Cogliati, M., A. Roverselli, et al. (1997). "Development of an in vitro macrophage system to assess *Penicillium marneffei* growth and susceptibility to nitric oxide." <u>Infection and immunity</u> **65**(1): 279-284.

Cooper, C. R. and N. Vanittanakom (2008). "Insights into the pathogenicity of *Penicillium marneffei*." <u>Future Microbiol</u> **3**(1): 43-55.

Cox, G. M., T. S. Harrison, et al. (2003). "Superoxide dismutase influences the virulence of *Cryptococcus neoformans* by affecting growth within macrophages." <u>Infect Immun</u> **71**(1): 173-180.

Cui, J., R. Tanaka, et al. (1997). "Histopathological and electron microscopical studies on experimental *Penicillium marneffei* infection in mice." <u>J Med Vet Mycol</u> **35**(5): 347-353.

Dang, Y., Q. Yang, et al. (2011). "RNA interference in fungi: pathways, functions, and applications." <u>Eukaryotic cell</u> **10**(9): 1148-1155.

Deng, Z., J. L. Ribas, et al. (1988). "Infections caused by *Penicillium marneffei* in China and Southeast Asia: review of eighteen published cases and report of four more Chinese cases." <u>Rev Infect Dis</u> **10**(3): 640-652.

Deng, Z. L. and D. H. Connor (1985). "Progressive disseminated penicilliosis caused by *Penicillium marneffei*. Report of eight cases and differentiation of the causative organism from Histoplasma capsulatum." <u>Am J Clin Pathol</u> **84**(3): 323-327.

Deng, Z. L., M. Yun, et al. (1986). "Human penicilliosis *marneffei* and its relation to the bamboo rat (*Rhizomys pruinosus*)." <u>J Med Vet Mycol</u> **24**(5): 383-389.

Didiano, D. and O. Hobert (2006). "Perfect seed pairing is not a generally reliable predictor for miRNA-target interactions." <u>Nature structural & molecular biology</u> **13**(9): 849-851.

Diederichs, S. and D. A. Haber (2007). "Dual role for argonautes in microRNA processing and posttranscriptional regulation of microRNA expression." <u>Cell</u> **131**(6): 1097-1108.

DiSalvo, A. F., A. M. Fickling, et al. (1973). "Infection caused by *Penicillium marneffei*: description of first natural infection in man." <u>Am J Clin Pathol</u> **60**(2): 259-263.

Drouhet, E. and P. Ravisse (1993). "Entomophthoromycosis." <u>Current topics in medical mycology</u> **5**: 215-245.

Duong, T. A. (1996). "Infection due to *Penicillium marneffei*, an emerging pathogen: review of 155 reported cases." <u>Clin Infect Dis</u> **23**(1): 125-130.

Eulalio, A., E. Huntzinger, et al. (2008). "GW182 interaction with Argonaute is essential for miRNA-mediated translational repression and mRNA decay." <u>Nature structural & molecular biology</u> **15**(4): 346-353.

Eulalio, A., E. Huntzinger, et al. (2009). "Deadenylation is a widespread effect of miRNA regulation." <u>RNA</u> **15**(1): 21-32.

Fairn, G. D. and C. R. McMaster (2008). "Emerging roles of the oxysterol-binding protein family in metabolism, transport, and signaling." <u>Cellular and molecular life sciences : CMLS</u> **65**(2): 228-236.

Fisher, M. C., W. P. Hanage, et al. (2005). "Low effective dispersal of asexual genotypes in heterogeneous landscapes by the endemic pathogen *Penicillium marneffei*." <u>PLoS Pathog</u> **1**(2): e20.

Friedlander, M. R., W. Chen, et al. (2008). "Discovering microRNAs from deep sequencing data using miRDeep." <u>Nature biotechnology</u> **26**(4): 407-415.

Fulci, V. and G. Macino (2007). "Quelling: post-transcriptional gene silencing guided by small RNAs in *Neurospora crassa*." <u>Current opinion in microbiology</u> **10**(2): 199-203.

Gellon, L., D. R. Carson, et al. (2008). "Intrinsic 5'-deoxyribose-5-phosphate lyase activity in *Saccharomyces cerevisiae* Trf4 protein with a possible role in base excision DNA repair." <u>DNA repair</u> **7**(2): 187-198.

Griffiths-Jones, S., R. J. Grocock, et al. (2006). "miRBase: microRNA sequences, targets and gene nomenclature." <u>Nucleic acids research</u> **34**(Database issue): D140-144.

Griffiths-Jones, S., H. K. Saini, et al. (2008). "miRBase: tools for microRNA genomics." <u>Nucleic acids research</u> **36**(Database issue): D154-158.

Grimson, A., K. K. Farh, et al. (2007). "MicroRNA targeting specificity in mammals: determinants beyond seed pairing." <u>Molecular cell</u> **27**(1): 91-105.

Guarnieri, D. J. and R. J. DiLeone (2008). "MicroRNAs: a new class of gene regulators." Annals of medicine **40**(3): 197-208.

Guarro, J., GeneJ, et al. (1999). "Developments in fungal taxonomy." Clinical microbiology reviews **12**(3): 454-500.

Gugnani, H., M. C. Fisher, et al. (2004). "Role of Cannomys badius as a natural animal host of *Penicillium marneffei* in India." J Clin Microbiol **42**(11): 5070-5075.

Guo, H. S., Q. Xie, et al. (2005). "MicroRNA directs mRNA cleavage of the transcription factor NAC1 to downregulate auxin signals for *Arabidopsis* lateral root development." Plant Cell **17**(5): 1376-1386.

Hafner, M., P. Landgraf, et al. (2008). "Identification of microRNAs and other small regulatory RNAs using cDNA library sequencing." Methods **44**(1): 3-12.

Haley, B. and P. D. Zamore (2004). "Kinetic analysis of the RNAi enzyme complex." Nature structural & molecular biology **11**(7): 599-606.

Hamilton, A. J., L. Jeavons, et al. (1999). "Recognition of fibronectin by *Penicillium marneffei* conidia via a sialic acid-dependent process and its relationship to the interaction between conidia and laminin." Infect Immun **67**(10): 5200-5205.

Hamilton, A. J., L. Jeavons, et al. (1998). "Sialic acid-dependent recognition of laminin by *Penicillium marneffei* conidia." Infect Immun **66**(12): 6024-6026.

Havecker, E. R., L. M. Wallbridge, et al. (2010). "The *Arabidopsis* RNA-directed DNA methylation argonautes functionally diverge based on their expression and interaction with target loci." The Plant cell **22**(2): 321-334.

Heath, T. C., A. Patel, et al. (1995). "Disseminated *Penicillium marneffei*: presenting illness of advanced HIV infection; a clinicopathological review, illustrated by a case report." Pathology **27**(1): 101-105.

Hibbett, D. S., M. Binder, et al. (2007). "A higher-level phylogenetic classification of the Fungi." Mycol Res **111**(Pt 5): 509-547.

Hilmarsdottir, I., J. L. Meynard, et al. (1993). "Disseminated *Penicillium marneffei* infection associated with human immunodeficiency virus: a report of two cases and a review of 35 published cases." J Acquir Immune Defic Syndr **6**(5): 466-471.

Hinas, A., J. Reimegard, et al. (2007). "The small RNA repertoire of *Dictyostelium discoideum* and its regulation by components of the RNAi pathway." Nucleic acids research **35**(20): 6714-6726.

Hoskins, I. C. and C. F. Roberts (1994). "Expression of the 3-phosphoglycerate kinase gene (pgkA) of *Penicillium chrysogenum*." Molecular & general genetics : MGG **243**(3): 270-276.

Hsueh, P. R., L. J. Teng, et al. (2000). "Molecular evidence for strain dissemination of *Penicillium marneffei*: an emerging pathogen in Taiwan." J Infect Dis **181**(5): 1706-1712.

Huh, W. K., S. T. Kim, et al. (2001). "Deficiency of D-erythroascorbic acid attenuates hyphal growth and virulence of *Candida albicans*." Infection and immunity **69**(6): 3939-3946.

Hulshof, C. M., R. A. van Zanten, et al. (1990). "*Penicillium marneffei* infection in an AIDS patient." Eur J Clin Microbiol Infect Dis **9**(5): 370.

Humphreys, D. T., B. J. Westman, et al. (2005). "MicroRNAs control translation initiation by inhibiting eukaryotic initiation factor 4E/cap and poly(A) tail function." Proceedings of the National Academy of Sciences of the United

States of America **102**(47): 16961-16966.

Huynh, T. X., H. C. Nguyen, et al. (2003). "[*Penicillium marneffei* infection and AIDS. A review of 12 cases reported in the Tropical Diseases Centre, Ho Chi Minh City (Vietnam)]." Sante **13**(3): 149-153.

Jack, T. (2004). "Molecular and genetic mechanisms of floral control." The Plant cell **16 Suppl**: S1-17.

Jahn, T. L., E. C. Bovee, et al. (1979). How to know the protozoa. Dubuque, Iowa, Wm. C. Brown Co.

Jakymiw, A., S. Lian, et al. (2005). "Disruption of GW bodies impairs mammalian RNA interference." Nat Cell Biol **7**(12): 1267-1274.

James, T. Y., F. Kauff, et al. (2006). "Reconstructing the early evolution of Fungi using a six-gene phylogeny." Nature **443**(7113): 818-822.

Jiang, N., Y. Yang, et al. (2012). "Identification and functional demonstration of miRNAs in the fungus *Cryptococcus neoformans*." PLoS One **7**(12): e52734.

Johnnidis, J. B., M. H. Harris, et al. (2008). "Regulation of progenitor cell proliferation and granulocyte function by microRNA-223." Nature **451**(7182): 1125-1129.

Johnson, S. M., H. Grosshans, et al. (2005). "RAS is regulated by the *let-7* microRNA family." Cell **120**(5): 635-647.

Jones, P. D. and J. See (1992). "*Penicillium marneffei* infection in patients infected with human immunodeficiency virus: late presentation in an area of nonendemicity." Clin Infect Dis **15**(4): 744.

Julander, I. and B. Petrini (1997). "*Penicillium marneffei* infection in a Swedish HIV-infected immunodeficient narcotic addict." Scand J Infect Dis **29**(3): 320-322.

Kadotani, N., H. Nakayashiki, et al. (2004). "One of the two Dicer-like proteins in the filamentous fungi *Magnaporthe oryzae* genome is responsible for hairpin RNA-triggered RNA silencing and related small interfering RNA accumulation." The Journal of biological chemistry **279**(43): 44467-44474.

Kaldor, J. M., W. Sittitrai, et al. (1994). "The emerging epidemic of HIV infection and AIDS in Asia and the Pacific." AIDS **8 Suppl 2**: S1-2.

Katiyar-Agarwal, S., R. Morgan, et al. (2006). "A pathogen-inducible endogenous siRNA in plant immunity." Proceedings of the National Academy of Sciences of the United States of America **103**(47): 18002-18007.

Kaufman, E. J. and E. A. Miska (2010). "The microRNAs of *Caenorhabditis elegans*." Seminars in cell & developmental biology **21**(7): 728-737.

Kavanagh, K. (2007). "New insights in medical mycology, Springer Netherlands: 304."

Kedde, M., M. J. Strasser, et al. (2007). "RNA-binding protein Dnd1 inhibits microRNA access to target mRNA." Cell **131**(7): 1273-1286.

Kendrick, B. (2000). "The fifth kingdom. New buryport Mass, Focus Pub: xii, 386."

Kendrick, B. (2001). The Fifth Kingdom, Focus Publishing/R. Pullins Company.

Kim, Y. K. and V. N. Kim (2007). "Processing of intronic microRNAs." The EMBO journal **26**(3): 775-783.

Kiriakidou, M., P. T. Nelson, et al. (2004). "A combined computational-experimental approach predicts human microRNA targets." Genes & development **18**(10): 1165-1178.

Kiriakidou, M., G. S. Tan, et al. (2007). "An mRNA m7G cap binding-like motif within

136

human Ago2 represses translation." Cell **129**(6): 1141-1151.

Krek, A., D. Grun, et al. (2005). "Combinatorial microRNA target predictions." Nature genetics **37**(5): 495-500.

Kronauer, C. M., G. Schar, et al. (1993). "[HIV-associated *Penicillium marneffei* infection]." Schweiz Med Wochenschr **123**(9): 385-390.

Kruger, J. and M. Rehmsmeier (2006). "RNAhybrid: microRNA target prediction easy, fast and flexible." Nucleic acids research **34**(Web Server issue): W451-454.

Kudeken, N., K. Kawakami, et al. (1996). "Cell-mediated immunity in host resistance against infection caused by *Penicillium marneffei*." Journal of medical and veterinary mycology : bi-monthly publication of the International Society for Human and Animal Mycology **34**(6): 371-378.

Kudeken, N., K. Kawakami, et al. (1997). "CD4+ T cell-mediated fatal hyperinflammatory reactions in mice infected with *Penicillium marneffei*." Clinical and experimental immunology **107**(3): 468-473.

Kudeken, N., K. Kawakami, et al. (1999). "Cytokine-induced fungicidal activity of human polymorphonuclear leukocytes against *Penicillium marneffei*." FEMS immunology and medical microbiology **26**(2): 115-124.

Kudeken, N., K. Kawakami, et al. (1999). "Role of superoxide anion in the fungicidal activity of murine peritoneal exudate macrophages against *Penicillium marneffei*." Microbiology and immunology **43**(4): 323-330.

Kudeken, N., K. Kawakami, et al. (2000). "Mechanisms of the in vitro fungicidal effects of human neutrophils against *Penicillium marneffei* induced by granulocyte-macrophage colony-stimulating factor (GM-CSF)." Clin Exp Immunol **119**(3): 472-478.

Kurihara, Y. and Y. Watanabe (2004). "*Arabidopsis* micro-RNA biogenesis through Dicer-like 1 protein functions." Proceedings of the National Academy of Sciences of the United States of America **101**(34): 12753-12758.

Lagos-Quintana, M., R. Rauhut, et al. (2001). "Identification of novel genes coding for small expressed RNAs." Science **294**(5543): 853-858.

Lagos-Quintana, M., R. Rauhut, et al. (2003). "New microRNAs from mouse and human." RNA **9**(2): 175-179.

Lagos-Quintana, M., R. Rauhut, et al. (2002). "Identification of tissue-specific microRNAs from mouse." Current biology : CB **12**(9): 735-739.

Lanet, E., E. Delannoy, et al. (2009). "Biochemical evidence for translational repression by *Arabidopsis* microRNAs." The Plant cell **21**(6): 1762-1768.

Lanford, R. E., E. S. Hildebrandt-Eriksen, et al. (2010). "Therapeutic silencing of microRNA-122 in primates with chronic hepatitis C virus infection." Science **327**(5962): 198-201.

Langmead, B., C. Trapnell, et al. (2009). "Ultrafast and memory-efficient alignment of short DNA sequences to the human genome." Genome biology **10**(3): R25.

Laniado-Laborin, R. (2007). "Coccidioidomycosis and other endemic mycoses in Mexico." Rev Iberoam Micol **24**(4): 249-258.

Lau, N. C., L. P. Lim, et al. (2001). "An abundant class of tiny RNAs with probable regulatory roles in *Caenorhabditis elegans*." Science **294**(5543): 858-862.

Lau, S. K., P. C. Woo, et al. (2012). "Isolation and characterization of a novel *Betacoronavirus* subgroup A coronavirus, rabbit coronavirus HKU14, from domestic rabbits." Journal of virology **86**(10): 5481-5496.

Lee, H. C., S. S. Chang, et al. (2009). "qiRNA is a new type of small interfering RNA induced by DNA damage." Nature **459**(7244): 274-277.

Lee, H. C., L. Li, et al. (2010). "Diverse pathways generate microRNA-like RNAs and Dicer-independent small interfering RNAs in fungi." Molecular cell **38**(6): 803-814.

Lee, R., R. Feinbaum, et al. (2004). "A short history of a short RNA." Cell **116**(2 Suppl): S89-92, 81 p following S96.

Lee, R. C. and V. Ambros (2001). "An extensive class of small RNAs in *Caenorhabditis elegans*." Science **294**(5543): 862-864.

Lee, R. C., R. L. Feinbaum, et al. (1993). "The *C. elegans* heterochronic gene *lin-4* encodes small RNAs with antisense complementarity to *lin-14*." Cell **75**(5): 843-854.

Lee, Y., C. Ahn, et al. (2003). "The nuclear RNase III Drosha initiates microRNA processing." Nature **425**(6956): 415-419.

Lee, Y., K. Jeon, et al. (2002). "MicroRNA maturation: stepwise processing and subcellular localization." The EMBO journal **21**(17): 4663-4670.

Lee, Y., M. Kim, et al. (2004). "MicroRNA genes are transcribed by RNA polymerase II." The EMBO journal **23**(20): 4051-4060.

Lee, Y. and V. N. Kim (2007). "In vitro and in vivo assays for the activity of Drosha complex." Methods in enzymology **427**: 89-106.

Lewis, B. P., C. B. Burge, et al. (2005). "Conserved seed pairing, often flanked by adenosines, indicates that thousands of human genes are microRNA targets." Cell **120**(1): 15-20.

Lim, L. P., M. E. Glasner, et al. (2003). "Vertebrate microRNA genes." Science **299**(5612): 1540.

Lim, L. P., N. C. Lau, et al. (2005). "Microarray analysis shows that some microRNAs downregulate large numbers of target mRNAs." Nature **433**(7027): 769-773.

Lin, C. A., S. R. Ellis, et al. (2010). "The Sua5 protein is essential for normal translational regulation in yeast." Molecular and cellular biology **30**(1): 354-363.

Liu, C. G., G. A. Calin, et al. (2004). "An oligonucleotide microchip for genome-wide microRNA profiling in human and mouse tissues." Proceedings of the National Academy of Sciences of the United States of America **101**(26): 9740-9744.

Liu, J., M. A. Carmell, et al. (2004). "Argonaute2 is the catalytic engine of mammalian RNAi." Science **305**(5689): 1437-1441.

Liu, J., M. A. Valencia-Sanchez, et al. (2005). "MicroRNA-dependent localization of targeted mRNAs to mammalian P-bodies." Nat Cell Biol **7**(7): 719-723.

Liu, N., S. Bezprozvannaya, et al. (2008). "microRNA-133a regulates cardiomyocyte proliferation and suppresses smooth muscle gene expression in the heart." Genes & development **22**(23): 3242-3254.

Lo, Y., K. Tintelnot, et al. (2000). "Disseminated *Penicillium marneffei* infection in an African AIDS patient." Trans R Soc Trop Med Hyg **94**(2): 187.

LoBuglio, K. F. and J. W. Taylor (1995). "Phylogeny and PCR identification of the human pathogenic fungus *Penicillium marneffei*." J Clin Microbiol **33**(1): 85-89.

Loftus, B. J., E. Fung, et al. (2005). "The genome of the basidiomycetous yeast and human pathogen *Cryptococcus neoformans*." Science **307**(5713): 1321-1324.

Low, K. a. S. S. L. (2002). "The pattern of AIDS Reporting and the implications on HIV surveillance." Public Health Epidemiol. Bull. **11**: 41-49.

Luh, K. T. (1998). "*Penicillium marneffei* fungemia in an AIDS patient: the first case report in Taiwan." Changgeng Yi Xue Za Zhi **21**(3): 362.

Lupi, O., S. K. Tyring, et al. (2005). "Tropical dermatology: fungal tropical diseases." J Am Acad Dermatol **53**(6): 931-951, quiz 952-934.

Lytle, J. R., T. A. Yario, et al. (2007). "Target mRNAs are repressed as efficiently by microRNA-binding sites in the 5' UTR as in the 3' UTR." Proceedings of the National Academy of Sciences of the United States of America **104**(23): 9667-9672.

Ma, J. B., Y. R. Yuan, et al. (2005). "Structural basis for 5'-end-specific recognition of guide RNA by the *A. fulgidus* Piwi protein." Nature **434**(7033): 666-670.

Mallory, A. and H. Vaucheret (2010). "Form, function, and regulation of ARGONAUTE proteins." The Plant cell **22**(12): 3879-3889.

Mallory, A. C., D. P. Bartel, et al. (2005). "MicroRNA-directed regulation of *Arabidopsis* AUXIN RESPONSE FACTOR17 is essential for proper development and modulates expression of early auxin response genes." The Plant cell **17**(5): 1360-1375.

Mallory, A. C., A. Hinze, et al. (2009). "Redundant and specific roles of the ARGONAUTE proteins AGO1 and ZLL in development and small RNA-directed gene silencing." PLoS genetics **5**(9): e1000646.

Mann, B., T. van Opijnen, et al. (2012). "Control of virulence by small RNAs in *Streptococcus pneumoniae*." PLoS pathogens **8**(7): e1002788.

Martinez, J., A. Patkaniowska, et al. (2002). "Single-stranded antisense siRNAs guide target RNA cleavage in RNAi." Cell **110**(5): 563-574.

Maselli, V., D. Di Bernardo, et al. (2008). "CoGemiR: a comparative genomics microRNA database." BMC genomics **9**: 457.

Mathonnet, G., M. R. Fabian, et al. (2007). "MicroRNA inhibition of translation initiation in vitro by targeting the cap-binding complex eIF4F." Science **317**(5845): 1764-1767.

Mattern, I., P. Punt, et al. (1988). "A vector of *Aspergillus* transformation conferring phleomycin resistance." Fungal Genet. Newsl **35**: 25.

McGuire, A. M. and J. E. Galagan (2008). "Conserved secondary structures in Aspergillus." PLoS One **3**(7): e2812.

Meister, G., M. Landthaler, et al. (2004). "Human Argonaute2 mediates RNA cleavage targeted by miRNAs and siRNAs." Molecular cell **15**(2): 185-197.

Meister, G., M. Landthaler, et al. (2005). "Identification of novel argonaute-associated proteins." Curr Biol **15**(23): 2149-2155.

Melton, C., R. L. Judson, et al. (2010). "Opposing microRNA families regulate self-renewal in mouse embryonic stem cells." Nature **463**(7281): 621-626.

mirbase. (2012). from http://www.mirbase.org.

Missall, T. A., J. K. Lodge, et al. (2004). "Mechanisms of resistance to oxidative and nitrosative stress: implications for fungal survival in mammalian hosts." Eukaryotic cell **3**(4): 835-846.

Molnar, A., F. Schwach, et al. (2007). "miRNAs control gene expression in the single-cell alga *Chlamydomonas reinhardtii*." Nature **447**(7148): 1126-1129.

Montgomery, T. A., M. D. Howell, et al. (2008). "Specificity of ARGONAUTE7-miR390 interaction and dual functionality in TAS3 trans-acting siRNA formation." Cell **133**(1): 128-141.

Mraz, M., D. Dolezalova, et al. (2012). "MicroRNA-650 expression is influenced by immunoglobulin gene rearrangement and affects the biology of chronic lymphocytic leukemia." Blood **119**(9): 2110-2113.

Mukherjee, K., H. Campos, et al. (2013). "Evolution of animal and plant dicers: early parallel duplications and recurrent adaptation of antiviral RNA binding in plants." Molecular biology and evolution **30**(3): 627-641.

Nakamura, K., A. Miyazato, et al. (2008). "Toll-like receptor 2 (TLR2) and dectin-1 contribute to the production of IL-12p40 by bone marrow-derived dendritic cells infected with *Penicillium marneffei*." Microbes and infection / Institut Pasteur **10**(10-11): 1223-1227.

Nakayashiki, H., S. Hanada, et al. (2005). "RNA silencing as a tool for exploring gene function in ascomycete fungi." Fungal Genet Biol **42**(4): 275-283.

Nakayashiki, H. and Q. B. Nguyen (2008). "RNA interference: roles in fungal biology." Current opinion in microbiology **11**(6): 494-502.

Nemecek, J. C., M. Wuthrich, et al. (2006). "Global control of dimorphism and virulence in fungi." Science **312**(5773): 583-588.

Nottrott, S., M. J. Simard, et al. (2006). "Human *let-7a* miRNA blocks protein production on actively translating polyribosomes." Nature structural & molecular biology **13**(12): 1108-1114.

Nykanen, A., B. Haley, et al. (2001). "ATP requirements and small interfering RNA structure in the RNA interference pathway." Cell **107**(3): 309-321.

O'Connell, R. M., K. D. Taganov, et al. (2007). "MicroRNA-155 is induced during the macrophage inflammatory response." Proceedings of the National Academy of Sciences of the United States of America **104**(5): 1604-1609.

O'Hara, S. P., J. L. Mott, et al. (2009). "MicroRNAs: key modulators of posttranscriptional gene expression." Gastroenterology **136**(1): 17-25.

Odling-Smee, L. (2007). "Complex set of RNAs found in simple green algae." Nature **447**(7144): 518.

Okamura, K., J. W. Hagen, et al. (2007). "The mirtron pathway generates microRNA-class regulatory RNAs in *Drosophila*." Cell **130**(1): 89-100.

Okamura, K., M. D. Phillips, et al. (2008). "The regulatory activity of microRNA* species has substantial influence on microRNA and 3' UTR evolution." Nature structural & molecular biology **15**(4): 354-363.

Olsen, P. H. and V. Ambros (1999). "The lin-4 regulatory RNA controls developmental timing in *Caenorhabditis elegans* by blocking LIN-14 protein synthesis after the initiation of translation." Developmental biology **216**(2): 671-680.

Ota, A., H. Tagawa, et al. (2004). "Identification and characterization of a novel gene, C13orf25, as a target for 13q31-q32 amplification in malignant lymphoma." Cancer research **64**(9): 3087-3095.

Palatnik, J. F., E. Allen, et al. (2003). "Control of leaf morphogenesis by microRNAs." Nature **425**(6955): 257-263.

Pallini, R., F. Pierconti, et al. (2001). "Evidence for telomerase involvement in the angiogenesis of astrocytic tumors: expression of human telomerase reverse transcriptase messenger RNA by vascular endothelial cells." Journal of neurosurgery **94**(6): 961-971.

Park, M. Y., G. Wu, et al. (2005). "Nuclear processing and export of microRNAs in *Arabidopsis*." Proceedings of the National Academy of Sciences of the United States of America **102**(10): 3691-3696.

Pasquinelli, A. E., B. J. Reinhart, et al. (2000). "Conservation of the sequence and temporal expression of *let-7* heterochronic regulatory RNA." Nature **408**(6808): 86-89.

Pautler, K. B., A. A. Padhye, et al. (1984). "Imported penicilliosis *marneffei* in the United States: report of a second human infection." Sabouraudia **22**(5): 433-438.

Perlman, D. C. and J. Carey (2006). "Prevention of Disseminated *Penicillium marneffei* in human immunodeficiency virus-infected Travelers." J Travel Med **13**(6): 386; author reply 387.

Petersen, C. P., M. E. Bordeleau, et al. (2006). "Short RNAs repress translation after initiation in mammalian cells." Molecular cell **21**(4): 533-542.

Peto, T. E., R. Bull, et al. (1988). "Systemic mycosis due to *Penicillium marneffei* in a patient with antibody to human immunodeficiency virus." J Infect **16**(3): 285-290.

Piehl, M. R., R. L. Kaplan, et al. (1988). "Disseminated penicilliosis in a patient with acquired immunodeficiency syndrome." Arch Pathol Lab Med **112**(12): 1262-1264.

Pillai, R. S., S. N. Bhattacharyya, et al. (2005). "Inhibition of translational initiation by Let-7 MicroRNA in human cells." Science **309**(5740): 1573-1576.

Pongpom, P., C. R. Cooper, Jr., et al. (2005). "Isolation and characterization of a catalase-peroxidase gene from the pathogenic fungus, *Penicillium marneffei*." Med Mycol **43**(5): 403-411.

Pratt, A. J. and I. J. MacRae (2009). "The RNA-induced silencing complex: a versatile gene-silencing machine." The Journal of biological chemistry **284**(27): 17897-17901.

Punt, P. J., R. P. Oliver, et al. (1987). "Transformation of *Aspergillus* based on the hygromycin B resistance marker from *Escherichia coli*." Gene **56**(1): 117-124.

Qi, Y., A. M. Denli, et al. (2005). "Biochemical specialization within *Arabidopsis* RNA silencing pathways." Molecular cell **19**(3): 421-428.

Rajagopalan, R., H. Vaucheret, et al. (2006). "A diverse and evolutionarily fluid set of microRNAs in *Arabidopsis thaliana*." Genes & development **20**(24): 3407-3425.

Ranjana, K. H., K. Priyokumar, et al. (2002). "Disseminated *Penicillium marneffei* infection among HIV-infected patients in Manipur state, India." J Infect **45**(4): 268-271.

Rehwinkel, J., I. Behm-Ansmant, et al. (2005). "A crucial role for GW182 and the DCP1:DCP2 decapping complex in miRNA-mediated gene silencing." RNA **11**(11): 1640-1647.

Reinhart, B. J., F. J. Slack, et al. (2000). "The 21-nucleotide *let-7* RNA regulates developmental timing in *Caenorhabditis elegans*." Nature **403**(6772): 901-906.

Reinhart, B. J., E. G. Weinstein, et al. (2002). "MicroRNAs in plants." Genes & development **16**(13): 1616-1626.

Rhoades, M. W., B. J. Reinhart, et al. (2002). "Prediction of plant microRNA targets."

Cell **110**(4): 513-520.

Robb, G. B. and T. M. Rana (2007). "RNA helicase A interacts with RISC in human cells and functions in RISC loading." Molecular cell **26**(4): 523-537.

Rodriguez, A., S. Griffiths-Jones, et al. (2004). "Identification of mammalian microRNA host genes and transcription units." Genome research **14**(10A): 1902-1910.

Rongrungruang, Y. and S. M. Levitz (1999). "Interactions of *Penicillium marneffei* with human leukocytes in vitro." Infection and immunity **67**(9): 4732-4736.

Ruby, J. G., C. Jan, et al. (2006). "Large-scale sequencing reveals 21U-RNAs and additional microRNAs and endogenous siRNAs in *C. elegans*." Cell **127**(6): 1193-1207.

Samson, R. A., N. Yilmaz, et al. (2011). "Phylogeny and nomenclature of the genus *Talaromyces* and taxa accommodated in *Penicillium* subgenus *Biverticillium*." Studies in mycology **70**(1): 159-183.

Sanchez-Martinez, C. and J. Perez-Martin (2001). "Dimorphism in fungal pathogens: Candida albicans and Ustilago maydis--similar inputs, different outputs." Curr Opin Microbiol **4**(2): 214-221.

Sanglard, D., F. Ischer, et al. (1996). "Susceptibilities of *Candida albicans* multidrug transporter mutants to various antifungal agents and other metabolic inhibitors." Antimicrob Agents Chemother **40**(10): 2300-2305.

Sar, B., S. Boy, et al. (2006). "In vitro antifungal-drug susceptibilities of mycelial and yeast forms of *Penicillium marneffei* isolates in Cambodia." J Clin Microbiol **44**(11): 4208-4210.

Sassen, S., E. A. Miska, et al. (2008). "MicroRNA: implications for cancer." Virchows Archiv : an international journal of pathology **452**(1): 1-10.

Schroder, K., P. J. Hertzog, et al. (2004). "Interferon-gamma: an overview of signals, mechanisms and functions." Journal of leukocyte biology **75**(2): 163-189.

Segers, G. C., X. Zhang, et al. (2007). "Evidence that RNA silencing functions as an antiviral defense mechanism in fungi." Proceedings of the National Academy of Sciences of the United States of America **104**(31): 12902-12906.

Seggerson, K., L. Tang, et al. (2002). "Two genetic circuits repress the *Caenorhabditis elegans* heterochronic gene *lin-28* after translation initiation." Developmental biology **243**(2): 215-225.

Segretain, G. (1959). "[*Penicillium marneffei* n.sp., agent of a mycosis of the reticuloendothelial system]." Mycopathologia **11**: 327-353.

Sen, G. L. and H. M. Blau (2005). "Argonaute 2/RISC resides in sites of mammalian mRNA decay known as cytoplasmic bodies." Nat Cell Biol **7**(6): 633-636.

Shibuya, K., S. Paris, et al. (2006). "Catalases of *Aspergillus fumigatus* and inflammation in aspergillosis." Nippon Ishinkin Gakkai Zasshi **47**(4): 249-255.

Sigova, A., N. Rhind, et al. (2004). "A single Argonaute protein mediates both transcriptional and posttranscriptional silencing in *Schizosaccharomyces pombe*." Genes & development **18**(19): 2359-2367.

Sirisanthana, T. and K. Supparatpinyo (1998). "Epidemiology and management of penicilliosis in human immunodeficiency virus-infected patients." Int J Infect Dis **3**(1): 48-53.

Sirisanthana, T., K. Supparatpinyo, et al. (1998). "Amphotericin B and itraconazole for treatment of disseminated *Penicillium marneffei* infection in human immunodeficiency virus-infected patients." <u>Clin Infect Dis</u> **26**(5): 1107-1110.

Slack, F. J., M. Basson, et al. (2000). "The *lin-41* RBCC gene acts in the *C. elegans* heterochronic pathway between the *let-7* regulatory RNA and the LIN-29 transcription factor." <u>Molecular cell</u> **5**(4): 659-669.

Sobottka, I., H. Albrecht, et al. (1996). "Systemic *Penicillium marneffei* infection in a German AIDS patient." <u>Eur J Clin Microbiol Infect Dis</u> **15**(3): 256-259.

Srinoulprasert, Y., P. Kongtawelert, et al. (2006). "Chondroitin sulfate B and heparin mediate adhesion of *Penicillium marneffei* conidia to host extracellular matrices." <u>Microb Pathog</u> **40**(3): 126-132.

Sun, Q., G. H. Choi, et al. (2009). "A single Argonaute gene is required for induction of RNA silencing antiviral defense and promotes viral RNA recombination." <u>Proceedings of the National Academy of Sciences of the United States of America</u> **106**(42): 17927-17932.

Supparatpinyo, K., S. Chiewchanvit, et al. (1992). "An efficacy study of itraconazole in the treatment of *Penicillium marneffei* infection." <u>J Med Assoc Thai</u> **75**(12): 688-691.

Supparatpinyo, K., S. Chiewchanvit, et al. (1992). "*Penicillium marneffei* infection in patients infected with human immunodeficiency virus." <u>Clin Infect Dis</u> **14**(4): 871-874.

Supparatpinyo, K., C. Khamwan, et al. (1994). "Disseminated *Penicillium marneffei* infection in southeast Asia." <u>Lancet</u> **344**(8915): 110-113.

Supparatpinyo, K., K. E. Nelson, et al. (1993). "Response to antifungal therapy by human immunodeficiency virus-infected patients with disseminated *Penicillium marneffei* infections and in vitro susceptibilities of isolates from clinical specimens." <u>Antimicrob Agents Chemother</u> **37**(11): 2407-2411.

Supparatpinyo, K. and H. T. Schlamm (2007). "Voriconazole as therapy for systemic *Penicillium marneffei* infections in AIDS patients." <u>Am J Trop Med Hyg</u> **77**(2): 350-353.

Takamizawa, J., H. Konishi, et al. (2004). "Reduced expression of the *let-7* microRNAs in human lung cancers in association with shortened postoperative survival." <u>Cancer research</u> **64**(11): 3753-3756.

Taramelli, D., S. Brambilla, et al. (2000). "Effects of iron on extracellular and intracellular growth of *Penicillium marneffei*." <u>Infection and immunity</u> **68**(3): 1724-1726.

Tavares, A. H., S. S. Silva, et al. (2005). "Virulence insights from the *Paracoccidioides brasiliensis* transcriptome." <u>Genet Mol Res</u> **4**(2): 372-389.

Thatcher, E. J., J. Bond, et al. (2008). "Genomic organization of zebrafish microRNAs." <u>BMC genomics</u> **9**: 253.

Thermann, R. and M. W. Hentze (2007). "*Drosophila miR2* induces pseudo-polysomes and inhibits translation initiation." <u>Nature</u> **447**(7146): 875-878.

Thirach, S., C. R. Cooper, Jr., et al. (2008). "Molecular analysis of the *Penicillium marneffei* glyceraldehyde-3-phosphate dehydrogenase-encoding gene (*gpdA*) and differential expression of gpdA and the isocitrate lyase-encoding gene (*acuD*) upon internalization by murine macrophages." <u>J Med Microbiol</u> **57**(Pt 11): 1322-1328.

Thirach, S., C. R. Cooper, Jr., et al. (2007). "The copper, zinc superoxide dismutase gene of *Penicillium marneffei*: cloning, characterization, and differential expression during phase transition and macrophage infection." Med Mycol **45**(5): 409-417.

Tsui, W. M., K. F. Ma, et al. (1992). "Disseminated *Penicillium marneffei* infection in HIV-infected subject." Histopathology **20**(4): 287-293.

UNAIDS (2007). "AIDS epidemic update 2007."

Ustianowski, A. P., T. P. Sieu, et al. (2008). "*Penicillium marneffei* infection in HIV." Curr Opin Infect Dis **21**(1): 31-36.

Valadi, H., K. Ekstrom, et al. (2007). "Exosome-mediated transfer of mRNAs and microRNAs is a novel mechanism of genetic exchange between cells." Nature cell biology **9**(6): 654-659.

Vanittanakom, N., C. R. Cooper, Jr., et al. (2006). "*Penicillium marneffei* infection and recent advances in the epidemiology and molecular biology aspects." Clin Microbiol Rev **19**(1): 95-110.

Vanittanakom, N., M. Mekaprateep, et al. (1995). "Efficiency of the flotation method in the isolation of *Penicillium marneffei* from seeded soil." J Med Vet Mycol **33**(4): 271-273.

Vaucheret, H., F. Vazquez, et al. (2004). "The action of ARGONAUTE1 in the miRNA pathway and its regulation by the miRNA pathway are crucial for plant development." Genes Dev **18**(10): 1187-1197.

Vaucheret, H., F. Vazquez, et al. (2004). "The action of ARGONAUTE1 in the miRNA pathway and its regulation by the miRNA pathway are crucial for plant development." Genes & development **18**(10): 1187-1197.

Vazquez, F., V. Gasciolli, et al. (2004). "The nuclear dsRNA binding protein HYL1 is required for microRNA accumulation and plant development, but not posttranscriptional transgene silencing." Curr Biol **14**(4): 346-351.

Viviani, M. A., A. M. Tortorano, et al. (1993). "Treatment and serological studies of an Italian case of penicilliosis *marneffei* contracted in Thailand by a drug addict infected with the human immunodeficiency virus." Eur J Epidemiol **9**(1): 79-85.

Wang, F., J. Tao, et al. (2009). "A histidine kinase PmHHK1 regulates polar growth, sporulation and cell wall composition in the dimorphic fungus *Penicillium marneffei*." Mycol Res **113**(Pt 9): 915-923.

Wang, Y. F., J. P. Cai, et al. (2011). "Immunoassays based on *Penicillium marneffei* Mp1p derived from Pichia pastoris expression system for diagnosis of penicilliosis." PLoS One **6**(12): e28796.

Wightman, B., I. Ha, et al. (1993). "Posttranscriptional regulation of the heterochronic gene *lin-14* by *lin-4* mediates temporal pattern formation in *C. elegans*." Cell **75**(5): 855-862.

Wong, K. H. and S. S. Lee (1998). "Comparing the first and second hundred AIDS cases in Hong Kong." Singapore Med J **39**(6): 236-240.

Wong, K. H., S. S. Lee, et al. (1998). "Redefining AIDS: case exemplified by *Penicillium marneffei* infection in HIV-infected people in Hong Kong." Int J STD AIDS **9**(9): 555-556.

Wong, L. P., P. C. Woo, et al. (2002). "DNA immunization using a secreted cell wall antigen Mp1p is protective against *Penicillium marneffei* infection." Vaccine

20(23-24): 2878-2886.

Wong, S. S., P. C. Woo, et al. (2001). "*Candida tropicalis* and *Penicillium marneffei* mixed fungaemia in a patient with Waldenstrom's macroglobulinaemia." <u>Eur J Clin Microbiol Infect Dis</u> **20**(2): 132-135.

Woo, P. C., K. T. Chong, et al. (2006). "Genomic and experimental evidence for a potential sexual cycle in the pathogenic thermal dimorphic fungus *Penicillium marneffei*." <u>FEBS Lett</u> **580**(14): 3409-3416.

Woo, P. C., C. W. Lam, et al. (2012). "First discovery of two polyketide synthase genes for mitorubrinic acid and mitorubrinol yellow pigment biosynthesis and implications in virulence of *Penicillium marneffei*." <u>PLoS neglected tropical diseases</u> **6**(10): e1871.

Woo, P. C., S. K. Lau, et al. (2011). "Draft genome sequence of *Penicillium marneffei* strain PM1." <u>Eukaryotic cell</u> **10**(12): 1740-1741.

Woo, P. C., E. W. Tam, et al. (2010). "High diversity of polyketide synthase genes and the melanin biosynthesis gene cluster in *Penicillium marneffei*." <u>FEBS J</u> **277**(18): 3750-3758.

Woo, P. C., H. Zhen, et al. (2003). "The mitochondrial genome of the thermal dimorphic fungus *Penicillium marneffei* is more closely related to those of molds than yeasts." <u>FEBS Lett</u> **555**(3): 469-477.

Wu, T. C., J. W. Chan, et al. (2008). "Clinical presentations and outcomes of *Penicillium marneffei* infections: a series from 1994 to 2004." <u>Hong Kong Med J</u> **14**(2): 103-109.

Xie, Z., K. D. Kasschau, et al. (2003). "Negative feedback regulation of Dicer-Like1 in *Arabidopsis* by microRNA-guided mRNA degradation." <u>Current biology : CB</u> **13**(9): 784-789.

Ye, X., N. Huang, et al. (2011). "Structure of C3PO and mechanism of human RISC activation." <u>Nature structural & molecular biology</u> **18**(6): 650-657.

Yi, R., Y. Qin, et al. (2003). "Exportin-5 mediates the nuclear export of pre-microRNAs and short hairpin RNAs." <u>Genes & development</u> **17**(24): 3011-3016.

Zhang, H., G. M. Ehrenkaufer, et al. (2013). "Small RNA pyrosequencing in the protozoan parasite *Entamoeba histolytica* reveals strain-specific small RNAs that target virulence genes." <u>BMC genomics</u> **14**(1): 53.

Zhang, H., F. A. Kolb, et al. (2004). "Single processing center models for human Dicer and bacterial RNase III." <u>Cell</u> **118**(1): 57-68.

Zheng, X., J. Zhu, et al. (2007). "Role of *Arabidopsis* AGO6 in siRNA accumulation, DNA methylation and transcriptional gene silencing." <u>The EMBO journal</u> **26**(6): 1691-1701.

Zhou, H. and K. Lin (2008). "Excess of microRNAs in large and very 5' biased introns." <u>Biochemical and biophysical research communications</u> **368**(3): 709-715.

Zhou, J., Y. Fu, et al. (2012). "Identification of microRNA-like RNAs in a plant pathogenic fungus *Sclerotinia sclerotiorum* by high-throughput sequencing." <u>Molecular genetics and genomics : MGG</u> **287**(4): 275-282.

Zhou, Q., M. Li, et al. (2012). "Immune-related microRNAs are abundant in breast milk exosomes." <u>International journal of biological sciences</u> **8**(1): 118-123.

Zhou, Q., Z. Wang, et al. (2012). "Genome-wide identification and profiling of microRNA-like RNAs from *Metarhizium anisopliae* during development."

Fungal biology **116**(11): 1156-1162.

Zhu, Q. H., A. Spriggs, et al. (2008). "A diverse set of microRNAs and microRNA-like small RNAs in developing rice grains." <u>Genome Res</u> **18**(9): 1456-1465.

Zilberman, D., X. Cao, et al. (2003). "ARGONAUTE4 control of locus-specific siRNA accumulation and DNA and histone methylation." <u>Science</u> **299**(5607): 716-719.

Zuber, S., M. J. Hynes, et al. (2002). "G-protein signaling mediates asexual development at 25 degrees C but has no effect on yeast-like growth at 37 degrees C in the dimorphic fungus *Penicillium marneffei*." <u>Eukaryotic cell</u> **1**(3): 440-447.

Zuber, S., M. J. Hynes, et al. (2003). "The G-protein alpha-subunit GasC plays a major role in germination in the dimorphic fungus *Penicillium marneffei*." <u>Genetics</u> **164**(2): 487-499.

CPSIA information can be obtained
at www.ICGtesting.com
Printed in the USA
BVOW05*1109080317
478099BV00002B/5/P